How to Look Young in Old Age:

Decoding the Science of Eternal Youth

By

Frank B. Trainer

Copyright © by Frank B. Trainer 2024. All rights reserved.

Before this document is duplicated or reproduced in any manner, the publisher's consent must be gained. Therefore, the contents within can neither be stored electronically, transferred, nor kept in a database. Neither in Part nor full can the document be copied, scanned, faxed, or retained without approval from the publisher or creator.

TABLE OF CONTENTS

Introduction

Aging:

Aging is a constant, endless process of natural change that starts in early childhood. During early middle age, several physical functions begin to gradually diminish. At the biological level, aging arises from the accumulation of a wide variety of molecular and cellular damage over time. This leads to a steady reduction in physical and mental capacity, a growing risk of disease, and ultimately death. These changes are neither linear nor consistent, and they are only weakly connected with a person's age in years. The variability exhibited in senior age is not random. Beyond biological changes, aging is typically connected with other life transitions such as retirement, moving to more fitting housing, and the death of friends and spouses. Aging is a phenomenon as ancient as time itself, yet one that has captivated humanity's curiosity for generations. It's a silent symphony that plays out throughout every cell of our being, a gradual dance with time that modifies our bodies and affects our experiences. Aging is the artwork of existence—the chapters that mark the passage of years and the progress of a lifetime.

But within the folds of time, there lives a common need—a shared yearning that transcends generations and countries—the yearning to keep the brilliance of youth even as the years approach.

Aging takes place in a cell, an organ, or a complete organism over time. It is a process that carries on during the entire adult life span of any living creature. Gerontology, the study of the aging process, is committed to the understanding and control of all variables contributing to the finitude of individual life. It is not concerned primarily with weakness, which looms so large in human experience but deals with a far larger spectrum of events. Every species has a life history in which the individual life span has an adequate relationship to the reproductive life span, the process of reproduction, and the path of development. How these associations formed is as pertinent to gerontology as it is to evolutionary biology. It is also vital to distinguish between the merely physicochemical processes of aging and the unintentional organismic processes of disease and injury that lead to mortality.

Gerontology, thus, might be described as the science of the finitude of life as manifested in the three elements of longevity, aging, and death, investigated from both evolutionary and individual (ontogenetic) perspectives. The term "old age" refers to the length of time that an organism has lived in its lifetime. Aging is the sequential or gradual change in an organism that leads to an increasing risk of debility, disease, and death. Senescence comprises various aspects of the aging process.

In a world that accepts diversity and champions the knowledge that accompanies age, the pull of youthfulness is as undeniable as the dawn's first light. It's in the sparkle of youthful eyes, the vigor of laughter, and the spring in each step. It's the cherished remembrance of carefree days and endless possibilities. Yet, behind the maze of science and sentiment, there is a paradox that has motivated humanity to examine the very essence of aging.

The Jewish tradition believes that old age is a continuation of the course that a person has chosen throughout their life until old age. A person does not change overnight; there is no rapid transition from 'young' to 'old' but rather, each person continues along a single route from youth to old age. Preparation for old age should begin while you are young. The more a person is aware of their mortality, the more they will be able to make the most of every moment and build up the abilities and attitudes that will offer them a pleasant old age. Agedness is a caution to prepare for death. This takes various forms: physical, economic, emotional, and spiritual. Preparing for death permits life to be lived to the utmost, without fear. It also creates the comfort and security of planning for an afterlife and existing beyond physical existence.

Even though the United States has an aging population, there is still a definite bias against aging and a general fear of being old. Even though the emphasis on youth and beauty has traditionally been aimed more toward females than males, we now see increased concern among males about aging and getting old. The elderly used to be a highly esteemed group and were valued for their experience and wisdom.

People do not become old or elderly at any set age. Traditionally, age 65 has been recognized as the beginning of old age. But the cause was rooted in history, not biology. Many years ago, age 65 was designated as the age for retirement in Germany, the first nation to create a retirement scheme. In 1965, in the United States, age 65 was selected as the eligibility age for Medicare insurance. This age is close to the real retirement age of most people in economically sophisticated cultures. **When a person turns elderly, this might be answered in several ways:**

• **Chronologic age** is based only on the passage of time. It is a person's age in years. Chronologic age has a defined importance in terms of health. Nonetheless, the likelihood of getting a health condition grows as people age, and it is health problems, rather than normal aging, that are the primary source of functional decline during old age. Because chronologic age can forecast numerous health problems, it has some legal and financial uses.

• **Biologic age** refers to changes in the body that usually occur as people age. These changes affect some people earlier than others, some people biologically get old at 65, and others do not until a decade or more later. However, most notable disparities in perceived age among people of identical chronologic age are produced by lifestyle, habit, and subtle impacts of disease rather than by variances in real aging.

• **Psychological age** is established by how people behave. For example, an 80-year-old who works, plans, looks forward to future events and participates in many activities is deemed psychologically younger.

Most healthy and active adults do not need the expertise of a geriatrician (a doctor who specializes in the care of elderly people) until they are 70, 75, or even 80 years old. However, some people need to see a geriatrician at a younger chronological age because of their medical issues.

Normal aging

People often question whether what they are feeling as they age is normal or odd. Although humans age somewhat differently, some changes arise from internal processes—that is, from aging itself. Hence, these changes are normal and called "pure aging." They occur universally in people who live long enough. the concept of pure aging. The modifications are to be expected and are generally unavoidable. For example, as people age, the lens of the eye swells, stiffens, and becomes less able to focus on close objects, such as reading materials (a disease called presbyopia).

This shift occurs in practically all elderly people. Thus, presbyopia is considered typical of aging. Other names used to describe these changes are "usual aging" and "senescence."

Exactly what constitutes normal aging is not always obvious. Changes that occur with normal aging render people more susceptible to developing certain illnesses. However, people can sometimes make efforts to adjust to these changes. As people get older, they become more susceptible to tooth loss. But seeing a dentist often, eating fewer sweets, and cleaning and flossing regularly may lower the odds of tooth loss. Thus, tooth loss, although common with aging, is an avoidable element of aging. Also, a functional decline that is part of aging sometimes seems similar to a functional decline that is part of a condition. For example, in senior age, a moderate reduction in mental performance is practically common and is called normal aging. This decline includes increasing difficulty learning new things, such as languages, a lower attention span, and increased forgetfulness. In comparison, the decline that occurs with dementia is substantially more severe.

People with normal aging may misplace things, while those with dementia forget entire events. People with dementia also have trouble executing routine daily chores (such as driving, cooking, and handling finances) and understanding the environment, including recognizing what year it is and where they are. Thus, dementia is considered a disorder, even if it is frequent later in life. Certain varieties of dementia, such as Alzheimer's disease, differ from normal aging in other ways as well. For example, brain tissue (obtained after autopsy) in people with Alzheimer's disease looks different from that in older people without the condition. So, the distinction between normal aging and dementia is evident. Sometimes, the boundary between functional decline, which is part of aging, and functional decline, which is part of an illness, seems arbitrary. For example, as people age, blood sugar levels climb more after ingesting carbs than they do in younger people. This rise is considered typical of aging. However, if the growth exceeds a specific level, diabetes, a condition, is identified. In this scenario, the difference is only one degree.

Healthy (successful) aging

Healthy aging refers to a postponement of or reduction in the unwanted effects of aging. The goals of healthy aging are maintaining physical and mental health, avoiding ailments, and remaining active and independent. For most people, maintaining general good health involves greater effort as they age. Certain healthy habits can be developed to improve overall well-being. Such as:

• Following a nutritious diet
• Avoiding cigarette smoking and heavy alcohol usage
• Exercising regularly
• Staying mentally active

The sooner a person develops these behaviors, the better. It's never too late to start. In this sense, people can have some control over what happens to them as they age.

Some data suggest that in the United States, healthy aging is on the rise.

• A drop in the percentage of adults aged 75 to 84 who report impairments
• A drop in the number of adults over 65 with debilitating diseases
• An increase in the elderly—people age 85 and older, including those who have reached 100 (centenarians)

Life Expectancy

The average life expectancy of Americans has been increasing considerably during the past century. A male child born in 1900 might expect to live only 46 years, and a female child, 48 years. In 2019, the average life expectancy in the US was 79 years for all people. Although much of this gain can be attributed to the large fall in juvenile mortality, life expectancy at every age beyond 40 has also grown dramatically. For example, a 65-year-old man can now expect to live to around age 83, and a 65-year-old woman to about age 86. Overall, women live around five years longer than men. This disparity in life expectancy has altered little, despite late 20th-century and early 21st-century changes in women's lifestyles, including smoking more and suffering greater stress.

Despite the increase in average life expectancy, the maximum life span—the oldest age to which humans can live—has changed little since records have been maintained. Despite the best genetic makeup and healthiest lifestyle, the possibility of living to be 120 is tiny. Madame Jeanne Calment had the longest reported lifespan: 122 years (1875–1997).

Several variables influence life expectancy, including:

• **Heredity:** Heredity impacts whether a person will acquire a disorder. For example, a person who inherits genes that enhance the likelihood of acquiring high cholesterol levels is likely to have a shorter life. A person with inherited protective genes against coronary heart disease and cancer may have a longer lifespan. There is solid evidence that living to a very long age—to 100 or older—runs in families.

• **Lifestyle:** Avoiding smoking, not abusing drugs and alcohol, maintaining a healthy weight and diet, exercising, and obtaining prescribed vaccines and screening examinations help people function well and avoid disorders.

• **Exposure to chemicals in the environment:** Such exposure can diminish life expectancy even among people with the best genetic composition.

• **Health care:** Preventing illnesses or treating disorders after they are contracted, especially where the disorder may be cured (as with infections and sometimes cancer), can enhance life expectancy.

This is where our trip begins.

In this book, "How to Look Young in Old Age: Decoding the Science of Eternal Youth," I will be disclosing the complicated code of aging. We shall examine the molecular symphonies that orchestrate the passage of time within our bodies, delving deep into the mechanisms that underpin the shift from youth to maturity. But beyond the scientific canvas, we uncover something fundamental: an undying longing that defies time itself.

As we journey through the chapters that follow, we'll explore not just the enigma of aging but the profound stories engraved into our hearts. We'll unearth the science underlying telomeres and DNA, the evolutionary dance that connects us to the rhythm of life, and the invisible footprints of time that show on the canvas of our skin. Yet, amongst this examination of science, we are also directed by a vision—a vision that looks beyond the lines engraved by age. A vision that integrates the cutting-edge findings of science with the practical art of everyday existence. The approach in this book is a unique blend of knowledge and action, where we attempt not simply to understand the symphony of aging but to master the art of guiding it.

We'll go through the epochs of time, exploring why we age, what causes our bodies to adapt, and how we can rewrite the tales of our aging. In each chapter, we'll reveal a new part of this ageless story, from the science of stem cells to the alchemy of nutrition, from the rhythms of exercise to the melodies of the mind. We'll investigate the secrets of epigenetics, decode the dialogues between our bodies and thoughts, and eventually design a blueprint for an ageless future.

This is a voyage of empowerment, a celebration of the beauty that develops with each passing year. As you turn the pages of this book, realize that you are not merely reading about science; you are embracing a vision, a philosophy, and a promise. I promise that age is not a number that defines us but a canvas upon which we paint our own stories of energy, wisdom, and timeless beauty. So, let us enter into the chapters that follow with hearts open and minds hungry for discovery. Let us expose the symphony of aging and, in doing so, change the way we look at the art of becoming older. Welcome to the voyage of a lifetime — a journey to unlock the science of eternal youth.

Chapter 1

The Mystery of Aging: Unraveling the Science Behind Aging

In the tapestry of life, there is a thread that weaves through time, a thread that carries with it the markings of years lived and stories told. This thread, this phenomenon we call aging, is both a masterpiece and a conundrum. It is a mystery that scientists and philosophers alike have struggled to decode for ages as they strive to fathom the secrets that lay within the very fabric of our being.

It is a known fact: we all age, and we all die. While no amount of science can change that, there is a chance scientists may be able to prevent, or at least slow down, the process of human aging amid a burst of new studies in this field. Many have been left convinced that healthy human lifespans can expand well beyond the existing limit of roughly 100 years, and this is due to the evolution of the human race. It has been previously asserted by scientists that there has been no advantage to humans living longer, with the major objective being to reproduce. This notion may certainly be obvious in the varied lifespans of humans compared to Giant Galapagos tortoises or Greenland sharks, who can live for around 300 years.

Aging is not just about beauty; it also bears the largest risk factor for diseases like Alzheimer's, heart disease, and cancer. While many of these cases are found in younger people, biologically, bodies grow less efficient at repair as they get older. This is why scientists are aiming to make additional substantial discoveries in the anti-aging sector. It might potentially halve the likelihood of humans developing these ailments and increase the average life expectancy by another notch. According to many experts, this is more than just a pipedream inspired by a science-fiction film and maybe a not-so-far-off reality, as there have already been some big achievements in this domain. And this is a field of scientific research that some of the world's richest entrepreneurs are taking an interest in.

$3 billion Amazon founder Jeff Bezos, for instance, sponsored anti-aging start-up Altos Labs with a hefty $3 billion (£2.5 billion) funding injection. And this is not Mr. Bezos' first effort in the anti-aging area either.

The billionaire has also injected funds into California-based firm UNITY Biotechnology, a start-up exploring medicines to halt or cure the effects of aging, with PayPal co-founder Peter Thiel also investing in the firm.

According to a survey by P&S Intelligence, the worldwide anti-aging industry is anticipated to jump from roughly £191.5 billion (£160 billion) at present levels to a startling $421.4 billion (£352 billion) by 2030.

Due to the massive financing the business is receiving, it is perhaps no surprise that interesting advances in the field are being uncovered more routinely. Bio Age is just one of those firms uncovering some amazing findings behind the secrets of aging.

Speaking about one of his major results, he described only one piece of study that may offer more substantial hints about life expectancy. He claimed it was a protein called apelin circulating in the blood, which seemed to make a difference. During the study, researchers found that middle-aged patients with higher levels of apelin in their blood tend to live longer. longer, with better muscle function and improved cognitive function as they age.

After being administered to very old mice, we proved that this medicine can enhance their muscle function. It made them go faster on their wheels; it increased their muscular size; it improved their grip strength." Now, a trial is beginning to investigate if the same medicine works as well in older humans in the same manner that it works for mice.

Scientists at the Salk Center for Biological Studies, a scientific research center in California, were also able to effectively reverse the aging process in middle-aged and old mice by partially resetting their cells to juvenile stages.

Known as cell rejuvenation therapy, the scientists at the Salk Institute employed reprogramming molecules to reset cells to more youthful states, making the mice's cells look younger. There was no increase in other health problems, including cancer.

Scientists are now monitoring the long-term effects of the therapy on animals, hoping to pave the way for future use in increasing...life expectancy of our species Juan Carlos, a professor in Salk's Gene Expression Laboratory, expressed his excitement about the potential of their approach to slow down aging in normal animals throughout their lifespan. The method has proven to be safe and efficient in mice This approach may offer a solution not only to age-related ailments but could also prove to be beneficial for the biomedical community. Our new tool improves cell function and resilience to restore tissue and organismal health in neurodegenerative diseases and other conditions.

Diving into the Molecular Undercurrents of Aging

At the heart of the enigma lies the intricate ballet of molecules and cells, a dance that orchestrates the passage of time within our bodies. Every breath we take, every heartbeat that echoes, is governed by these molecular choreographies. The science of aging seeks to unveil these choreographies and comprehend the mechanisms that shape the transitions from youth to maturity. Within our cells, a world unfolds. Telomeres, those delicate caps at the ends of our chromosomes, stand as sentinels against the march of time. These protective shields guard our genetic information, like the bookmarks of life's chapters. But as the pages of time turn, telomeres erode, much like the wax of a candle flickers away.

This erosion, like the ticking of a cosmic clock, plays a role in dictating our lifespan.

Unraveling the Role of Telomeres, DNA Damage, and Cellular Senescence

Recent research indicates that telomere length, which can be influenced by different lifestyle factors, can affect the pace of aging and the onset of age-associated illnesses. Telomeres are structures made up of DNA and protein that are located at the end of chromosomes. They prevent degradation, recombination, and fusion. Telomeres have a crucial function in safeguarding the integrity of the genetic material in our cells. Telomeres play a crucial role in protecting the integrity of our genetic material. When telomere length reaches a critical limit, the cell undergoes senescence and/or apoptosis Telomere length can function as a biological clock determining a cell's lifespan. an organism. Certain lifestyle factors may cause damage to the telomeres, leading to faster telomere shortening. to DNA in general or, more specifically, at telomeres and may, therefore, affect the health and lifespan of an individual.

In this review, we highlight the lifestyle factors that may adversely affect the health and lifespan of an individual by accelerating telomere shortening and also those that can potentially Protect telomeres is crucial for maintaining an individual's health.

The structure and functions of telomeres

Telomeres, the DNA-protein complexes at chromosome ends, protect the genome from degradation and interchromosomal fusion. Telomeric DNA is associated with telomere-binding proteins, and a loop structure mediated by TRF2 protects the ends of human chromosomes against exonucleolytic degradation and may also prime telomeric DNA The process involves synthesizing missing DNA segments through a mechanism that is comparable to 'gap filling' in homologous recombination. As shown, telomere shortening occurs at each DNA replication and, if continued, leads to chromosomal degradation and cell death. Telomerase activity, which extends telomeres, is present in germline and some hematopoietic cells. Somatic cells have low or undetectable levels of activity. undergo a progressive shortening with replication.

Telomerases are enzymes that are commonly reactivated in cancerous cells and immortalized cells, leading to their immortality and proliferation. A specific group of cells that have either undergone immortalization or turned cancerous do not possess the ability to produce telomerase, yet they are able to sustain the length of their telomeres.by alternative mechanisms, probably involving genetic (homologous) recombination, which is elevated in most immortal/cancer cell lines. We have found that telomerase physically interacts with the recombinase family of proteins and inhibitors of homologous recombination, reducing telomere length in telomerase-positive Barrett's adenocarcinoma cells (unpublished data from our laboratory). It is suggested that recombinational repair is closely associated with the maintenance of telomeres.

Telomere shortening and the aging process

Telomeres shrink with age, and the rate of telomere shortening may indicate the pace of aging. Telomere length reduces with age and may predict your longevity. Normal diploid cells have a limited lifespan in culture because they lose telomeres with each cell division.

Human liver tissues lose 55 telomeric DNA base pairs per year. The rate of telomere shortening in rapidly renewing gastric mucosal cells is similar to that observed. Liver tissue. Stathmin and EF-1a are biomarkers that indicate telomeric dysfunction and DNA damage, respectively. In a cell, increase with age and age-related diseases in humans Age correlates negatively with telomere length and positively with p16 expression, which increases in aging cells.

Accelerated telomere shortening in the genetic disorder dyskeratosis congenital is associated with the early onset of several age-associated disorders and a reduced lifespan. Telomerase activity, the ability to add telomeric repeats to the chromosome ends, is present in germline, hematopoietic, stem, and certain other rapidly renewing cells but is extremely low or absent in most normal somatic cells. The introduction of a telomerase gene through transgenic methods in normal human cells has been observed to extend their lifespan. Cawthon et al. showed that individuals with shorter telomeres had significantly poorer survival due to higher mortality rates caused by heart and infectious diseases.

The gradual reduction in the length of telomeres ultimately results in cellular senescence, apoptotic cell death, or oncogenic transformation. of somatic cells in various tissues. Telomere length, influenced by lifestyle, impacts lifespan and health., and the rate at which an individual is aging.

Telomeres, which are essential components of our chromosomes, naturally shorten as we age. Telomere length in humans decreases 24.8-27.7 base pairs annually.Telomere length, which is shorter than the average telomere length for a specific age group, has been associated with an increased incidence of age-related diseases and/or a decreased lifespan in humans. Telomere length is affected by a combination of factors, including donor age, genetic and epigenetic makeup and environment, social and economic status, exercise, body weight, and smoking Gender does not have a significant effect on telomere loss rate. When the length of telomeres shortens beyond a certain threshold, it triggers a process of cellular senescence and/or programmed cell death, known as apoptosis.

Certain lifestyle factors, such as smoking, obesity, lack of exercise, and consumption of an unhealthy diet, can increase the pace of telomere shortening, leading to illness and/or premature death. The early onset of many age-related health issues is often linked to accelerated telomere shortening. problems, including coronary heart disease, heart failure, diabetes, increased cancer risk, and osteoporosis. Individuals whose leukocyte telomeres are shorter than the corresponding average telomere length have a three-fold higher risk of developing myocardial infarction. Evaluation of telomere length in elders shows that individuals with shorter telomeres have a much higher rate of mortality than those with longer telomeres Excessive or accelerated telomere shortening can have negative impacts on health and lifespan across various levels. Shorter telomeres can also induce genomic instability by mediating interchromosomal fusion and may contribute to telomere stabilization and the development of cancer. Telomerase activity is typically higher in cancer cells, while telomere length is shorter. relative to corresponding control cells.

We found that cancer cell lines and primary cancer cells have shorter telomere lengths, as shown by laser capture microdissection. However, inhibition of telomere maintenance mechanisms and continued telomere shortening induce senescence and/or apoptosis in immortal and cancer cells.

Shorter telomeres have been identified as a risk factor for cancer, according to various studies. Individuals with shorter telomeres seem to have a greater risk of developing lung, bladder, renal cell, gastrointestinal, and head and neck cancers. Certain individuals may also be born with shorter telomeres or may have a genetic disorder leading to shorter telomeres. Such individuals are at a greater risk of developing premature coronary heart disease and premature aging. Deficiency of the telomerase RNA gene in a genetic disorder called dyskeratosis congenital leads to shorter telomeres and is associated with premature graying, a predisposition to cancer, vulnerability to adults may experience infections, as well as progressive bone marrow failure, which can lead to premature death.

Effects of smoking and obesity on telomeres and aging

Smoking and obesity tend to have an unfavorable influence on telomeres and aging. Smoking may speed up the telomere shortening and aging processes.

Excessive shortening of telomeres can cause genomic instability and can also lead to the development of tumors. Cancer cells typically exhibit shorter telomeres compared to normal cells. Smoking is associated with accelerated telomere shortening. Cancer cells often have shorter telomeres than normal cells. Smoking can increase the rate of telomere shortening, which may contribute to the development of cancer. A dose-dependent increase in telomere shortening has been observed in the blood cells of tobacco smokers. A study conducted in the white blood cells of women indicates that telomeric DNA is lost at an average rate of 25.7–27.7 base pairs per year, and with daily smoking of each pack of cigarettes, an additional five base pairs are lost. Smoking one pack of cigarettes a day for 40 years causes telomere attrition equivalent to 7.4 years of life. Babizhayev et al. It has been proposed that telomere length can be used as a biomarker to evaluate oxidative damage.ge caused by smoking and may also predict the rate at which an individual is aging.

It has been suggested that telomere length may serve as a biomarker for evaluating oxidative damage. antioxidant therapy. In summary, smoking increases oxidative stress expedites telomere shortening, and may increase the pace of the aging process.

Obesity is linked to higher levels of oxidative stress and DNA damage. Furukawa et al. showed that waist circumference and BMI significantly correlate with elevated plasma and urinary levels of reactive oxygen species. Song et al. Studies have indicated that body mass index (BMI) is strongly associated with biomarkers of DNA damage, regardless of age. The increased oxidative stress associated with obesity is likely caused by an irregular production of adipocytokines. Obese KKAy mice display higher plasma levels of reactive oxygen species and lipid peroxidation relative to control C57BL/6 mice The white adipose tissue of obese mice showed elevated levels of reactive oxygen species. But not in other tissues, indicating that the oxidative stress detected in plasma The production of oxidizing agents in the fat tissue could be the reason behind this.

Moreover, the transcript levels and activities of antioxidant enzymes, including catalase and dismutase, were significantly lower in the white adipose tissue of obese mice relative to control mice. The authors propose that a lack of antioxidant defense and an elevated NADPH oxidase pathway in accrued fat probably led to increased oxidative stress in obese animals. Exposure to oxidative stress can cause damage to DNA, which in turn can accelerate the shortening of telomeres. Telomeres in obese women are significantly shorter than those in lean women of the same age group. The excessive loss of telomeres in obese individuals was calculated to be equivalent to 8.8 years of life, an effect that seems to be worse than smoking. Together, these data indicate that obesity hurts telomeres and may unnecessarily expedite the process of aging.

Effects of environment, kind of employment, and stress on telomeres and aging

Environment, kind of career, and stress can also affect the pace of telomere shortening and health.
Hoxha et al.

The study assessed the length of telomeres in the white blood cells of both office workers and traffic police officers exposed to traffic pollution. The levels of toluene and benzene were used to indicate the extent of pollution exposure The telomere length of traffic police officers was found to be shorter within each age group by the investigators relative to telomere length in office workers. The lymphocytes of coke-oven workers who were exposed to polycyclic aromatic hydrocarbons also showed similar effects significantly shorter telomeres and increased evidence of DNA damage and genetic instability relative to control subjects. Although the reduction in telomere length in these workers did not correlate with age or markers of DNA damage, it significantly correlated with the number of years the workers were exposed to harmful agents. Telomere attrition has been associated with increased cancer risk, and coke-oven workers are at a greater risk of developing lung cancer. As we age, the shortening of telomeres in lymphocytes is also observed.

Consistently, the reduced telomere length in the lymphocytes of coke-oven workers was also associated with hypomethylation of the p53 promoter, which may induce the expression of p53, leading to inhibition of growth or induction of apoptosis. Thus, exposure to genotoxic agents, which may induce damage to DNA in general or more extensively at telomeres, can increase cancer risk and the pace of aging.

Stress leads to the secretion of glucocorticoid hormones by the adrenal gland. Let me know if you want me to make any further changes. Research has shown that these hormones can decrease levels of antioxidant proteins, potentially impacting health., cause increased oxidative damage to DNA and accelerated telomere shortening. Consistently, the women exposed to stress in their daily lives had evidence of increased oxidative pressure, reduced telomerase activity, and shorter telomeres in peripheral blood mononuclear cells relative to the women in the control group. Importantly, the difference in telomere length in these two groups of women was equivalent to 10 years of life, indicating that the women under stress were at risk for the early onset of age-related health problems.

Because telomere length may indicate an individual's biological age, stress would adversely affect health and longevity.

Effects of nutrition, dietary restrictions, and exercise on telomeres and aging

What we eat and how much we eat can dramatically affect our telomeres, health, and longevity. Let's look at the impact of fiber, fat, and protein on telomeres and aging. Cassidy et al. After analyzing a large sample, we studied how lifestyle factors relate to leukocyte telomere length group of women. Telomere length correlates positively with fiber intake and negatively with waist circumference and intake of polyunsaturated fatty acids - particularly linoleic acid. A reduction in protein intake from food also seems to increase longevity. A reduction in the protein content of food by 40% led to a 15% increase in the lifespan of rats. The rats that were fed a protein-restricted diet during early stages of life displayed long-term suppression of appetite., reduced growth rate, and increased lifespan, and the increased lifespan in such animals The study found that the kidney was linked with longer telomeres.

Consistently, the highest life expectancy of Japanese is associated with low protein and high-carbohydrate intake in the diet. The source of protein also seems to be an important factor, as replacing casein with soy protein in rats is associated with a delayed incidence of chronic nephropathies and an increased lifespan.

Dietary consumption of antioxidants reduces the rate of telomere shortening.

A study by Farzaneh-Far et al. Consuming a diet rich in antioxidant omega-3 fatty acids is linked to reduced telomere shortening, whereas a deficiency in these antioxidants is linked to increased shortening. of telomere attrition in study participants. The authors tracked omega-3 levels in blood and telomere length. a period of 5 years and found an inverse correlation, indicating that antioxidants reduce the rate of telomere shortening. Similarly, the women who consumed a diet lacking antioxidants had shorter telomeres and a moderate risk for the development of breast cancer, whereas the consumption of a diet rich in antioxidants such as vitamin E, vitamin C, and beta-carotene was associated with longer telomeres and a lower risk of breast cancer.

Antioxidants have the potential to protect telomeric DNA from oxidative damage that is caused by external factors. intrinsic DNA-damaging agents.

Dietary restriction lowers the pace of aging.

Restricting the amount of food you consume, also known as dietary restriction, can have a significantly positive impact on your health and lifespan. Reducing food intake in animals leads to a reduced growth rate, reduced oxidative burden, and reduced damage to DNA, which, therefore, keeps the animals in a biologically younger state A healthy lifestyle can significantly extend one's lifespan by up to 66%. Restricting rodents' diet delays age-related diseases onset. and increases the lifespan. Rats that were given a diet low in protein during early development showed a long-term decrease in appetite. a reduced growth rate, and an increased lifespan. The study found that the presence of this particular factor was linked to longer telomeres in the kidneys. Because oxidative stress can substantially accelerate telomere shortening, the reduction in oxidative stress caused by dietary restriction is expected to preserve telomeres and other cellular components.

Exercise may protect telomeres and slow the process of aging.

Song et al. have demonstrated that the duration of exercise inversely correlates with biomarkers for damage to DNA and telomeres and with p16 expression, a biomarker for aging human cells. Exercise can reduce harmful fat and promote waste elimination. reduced oxidative stress and preservation of DNA and telomeres. Werner et al. A study demonstrated that regular exercise is linked to increased telomerase activity and the inhibition of various factors. apoptosis proteins, including p53 and p16, in mice. Consistently, in humans, the leukocytes derived from athletes had elevated telomerase activity and reduced telomere shortening relative to non-athletes. Exercise seems to be associated with reduced oxidative stress and elevated expression of telomere-stabilizing proteins, which may therefore. Reduce the pace of aging and age-associated diseases.

In recap, telomeres shorten with age, and progressive telomere shortening leads to senescence and/or apoptosis. Shorter telomeres have also been implicated in genomic instability and oncogenesis.

Older people with shorter telomeres have a three- and eight-fold increased risk of dying from heart disease and infectious diseases, respectively. The rate of telomere shortening is, therefore, critical to an individual's health and pace of aging. Exposure to pollution, smoking, lack of physical activity, obesity, stress, and an unhealthy diet increase health risks. the oxidative burden and the rate of telomere shortening. To preserve telomeres and reduce cancer risk and the pace of aging, we may consider eating less, including antioxidants, fiber, soy protein, and healthy fats (derived from avocados, fish, and nuts) in our diet, and staying lean, active, healthy, and stress-free through regular exercise and meditation. Foods such as tuna, salmon, herring, mackerel, halibut, anchovies, catfish, grouper, flounder, flax seeds, chia seeds, sesame seeds, kiwi, black raspberries, lingonberry, green tea, broccoli, sprouts, red grapes, tomatoes, Foods such as olives, rich in vitamin C and vitamin E, serve as excellent providers of antioxidants.

These, combined with a Mediterranean-type diet containing fruits and whole grains, would help protect telomeres.

Telomeres are not the only players in this complex symphony. DNA damage, caused by a lifetime of exposure to various stressors, can accumulate over the years. Our cells are remarkably adept at repairing this damage, but as time goes on, the repair mechanisms may falter. Like cracks forming in a once-solid foundation, this DNA damage can contribute to the aging process. Cellular senescence, another crucial element, involves cells entering a state of dormancy and no longer actively dividing. While this state can protect us from damaged cells that might otherwise cause harm, it also contributes to the overall decline of tissue function. These senescent cells, once beneficial, can become a double-edged sword as they accumulate.

Biological Age vs. Chronological Age: Unveiling the Rift

Imagine a world where our age is not defined solely by the years, we've lived but by the state of our cells, the vitality of our bodies, and the resilience of our minds. This is the world of the biological age.

While chronological age counts the years since our birth, biological age factors in the wear and tear on our bodies, the strength of our immune systems, and the overall health of our cells.

The concept of biological age challenges the traditional notion of aging as a linear process. Instead, it paints a dynamic portrait of our bodies as they respond to the influences of genetics, lifestyle, and environment. This shift in perspective has far-reaching implications, from redefining our understanding of health to inspiring new avenues for intervention.

The Tapestry of Aging: A Story Continuously Unfolding

As we delve into the molecular depths of aging, we uncover a story of complexity, resilience, and transformation. Telomeres whisper tales of time's passage, DNA damage tells of battles waged, and cellular senescence hints at a delicate balance between protection and decline. The concept of biological age presents a new lens through which to view the chapters of our lives, inviting us to rewrite our stories with the ink of science and the brushstrokes of action.

In the chapters that follow, we'll explore how this science can be harnessed and how the threads of molecular dance can be steered toward vitality and rejuvenation. But as we step into this realm of discovery, let us not forget the wonder that accompanies each sunrise and sunset, the beauty that emerges in the laughter lines and silver strands. For within the enigma of aging lies a truth that defies time itself—the truth that our journey is both a puzzle to be solved and a masterpiece to be celebrated.

Chapter 2

The Clock of Life: Why We Age

Aging does not come all of a sudden. Instead, it's a constant biological process that accompanies us throughout our lives, beginning when we are born and ending when we die. Due to the progress of medical techniques and the enhancement of hygienic circumstances, the human lifespan has virtually doubled during the last 120 years.

Aging ranks with sleep as one of the primary mysteries of human biology. What causes the body to slow down, its cells to stop dividing and its organs to fall prey to increasing sickness and disability? No one has definitive answers to these issues, but theories can be classified into two camps: progressive harm over time and genetic programming.

The first group of beliefs says that the body ages due to wear and tear that builds in the tissues throughout the years. Waste products pile up in cells, backup systems fail, repair mechanisms gradually break down, and the body just wears out like an old automobile.

The second group thinks that aging is driven by our genes—by an internal molecular clock set to a particular timetable for each species. Support for this notion comes from animal studies: Scientists have been able to produce an enhanced life span in some animals by tweaking just one gene. Biologists point out that, from an evolutionary point of view, the impacts of natural selection drastically reduce after reproductive age. Evolution promotes genes that are useful early in life, directing the body's resources into reproduction and leaving them less accessible for long-term upkeep.

Theories on aging

It's generally believed that aging is caused by numerous processes rather than one explanation. It's also possible that these processes interact and overlap with each other. Below are some of the most important theories of aging:

Programmed theories of aging

Programmed aging ideas state that individuals are created to age and that our cells have a predetermined lifespan that's encoded into our bodies.

Also dubbed active, or adaptive, aging theories, they include:

• **Gene theory:** This idea claims that specific genes turn "on" and "off" over time, causing aging.

• **Endocrine hypothesis**: According to this idea, aging is caused by changes in hormones, which are produced by the endocrine system.

• **The immunological theory, also dubbed the autoimmune theory:** is the belief that the immune response is supposed to diminish. The result is sickness and aging.

Programmed theories have many proponents. However, they imply that activities linked to lifespan, such as quitting smoking and exercising, are ineffective. This is likely erroneous, as research has constantly demonstrated that certain habits decrease life expectancy.

Error ideas of aging

Error theories, or damage theories, are the antithesis of programmed theories. They propose that aging is driven by cellular changes that are random and unplanned.

Error theories of aging include:

• **Wear and tear hypothesis:** This is the belief that cells break down and get damaged over time. But critics contend that it doesn't account for the body's ability to mend.

• **Genome instability theory**: According to this idea, aging happens because the body loses its ability to repair DNA damage.

• **Cross-linkage theory:** This theory states that aging is due to the development of cross-linked proteins, which damage cells and hinder biological functioning.

• **Rate-of-living theory:** Proponents of this hypothesis claim that an organism's rate of metabolism affects its longevity. However, the notion lacks significant and consistent scientific proof.

• **Free radical theory**: This idea says that aging is related to the development of oxidative stress, which is caused by free radicals. However, some argue this idea fails to explain other types of cellular damage seen in aging.

• **Mitochondrial hypothesis:** as a version of the free radical theory, this theory states that mitochondrial damage releases free radicals and causes aging. The theory lacks hard scientific evidence.

The genetic theory of aging

The genetic theory claims that aging mostly depends on genetics. In other words, our life expectancy is determined by the genes we acquire from our parents. Since genes have predefined traits, it's thought that this idea coincides with programmed views of aging. Genetic theories include:

• **Telomere hypothesis:** Telomeres preserve the ends of your chromosomes as they multiply. Over time, telomeres shrink, which is connected with disease and aging.

• **programmed senescence theory:** Cellular senescence happens when cells stop reproducing and developing but don't die. This idea says that this causes aging.

• **Stem cell theory:** stem cells can change into different cells, which helps heal tissue and organs. However, the function of stem cells reduces over time, potentially contributing to aging.

• **Longevity gene theory:** This is the theory that certain genes enhance lifespan. More research is essential. Longevity genes, those uncommon riches carried by some humans, confer the gift of extended life. But genetics are not just about lifespans.

They also influence how we age, impacting aspects such as the rate at which our cells deteriorate and our vulnerability to certain age-related diseases.

The problem with genetic theories is that they neglect the importance of extrinsic influences. In contrast, it's estimated that just 25 percent of trusted sources of longevity are determined by heredity. This shows that environmental and behavioral variables have a crucial impact.

Evolutionary theory of aging

Natural selection refers to the adaptive features of an organism. These features can assist the organism in adjusting to its environment, so they're more likely to survive.

According to evolutionary theories, aging is based on natural selection. It argues that an organism begins aging when it has reached its peak of reproduction and has passed down adaptive features.

Evolutionary hypotheses include:

• **Mutation accumulation:** This theory posits that random mutations accumulate during the later stages of life.

• **Antagonistic pleiotropy:** According to this notion, genes that enhance fertility early in life have deleterious impacts later on.

• **Disposable soma theory:** The theory suggests that when more metabolic resources are devoted toward reproduction, less is spent on DNA repair. This leads to cellular damage and the aging process.

Evolutionary theories imply that aging, in some settings, serves a purpose. In the larger picture of species survival, the allocation of resources towards the young can ensure their prospects of survival and dissemination. This notion is obvious in animals, where longevity is tightly tied to reproduction. But this is just one brushstroke on the canvas of a complicated evolutionary portrait.

These possibilities are still being investigated and require further evidence.

The biochemical theory of aging

Another theory is that biological reactions cause aging. These reactions occur naturally and continually throughout life.

This hypothesis is rooted in numerous principles, including:

• **Advanced glycation end products (AGEs):** AGEs form when lipids or proteins are exposed to sugar. High amounts may lead to oxidative stress, which speeds up aging.

• **Heat shock reaction:** Heat shock proteins protect cells from stress, but their reaction weakens as we age.

• **Damage buildup:** Normal chemical reactions destroy DNA, proteins, and metabolites over time.

The Symphony of Lifestyle, Environment, and Inflammation

The theater upon which our lives unfold is not confined to genetics alone. Lifestyle choices such as smoking and excessive alcohol use, environmental effects such as air pollution, and the symphony of inflammation intermingle to construct the narrative of aging. Our choices, from the foods we consume to our exercise regimens, can tip the balance between youthful energy and hastened decline. Environmental stressors, ranging from pollution to UV radiation, throw shadows over our cellular canvases, leading to the obvious indicators of aging.

Meanwhile, inflammation, generally considered a double-edged sword, bears ramifications beyond its involvement in the immune response. Chronic inflammation, induced by causes such as stress and a poor diet, can accelerate cellular degeneration and contribute to the aging process.

Chapter 3

The Fountain of Youth: Unlocking the Anti-Aging Toolbox

Within the folds of time is a quest that spans generations: the quest for the mythical Fountain of Youth. As science moves forward, unearthing the mysteries of the human body, we stand on the cusp of an era that may see the borders of aging redefined. This chapter digs into a realm of possibilities where science transforms into alchemy, presenting a comprehensive arsenal that questions the very essence of aging.

Crafting an Arsenal Against Aging: A Comprehensive Toolkit

Imagine a toolkit stocked with precision equipment designed to disassemble the mechanics of aging, piece by delicate component. This toolset is a symphony of science and creativity, a harmony of discoveries aimed at breaking the conventional boundaries of our lives. It comprises a vast diversity of techniques, each poised to intercept the aging process at its source.

The Marvel of Stem Cells and Regenerative Medicine as An Anti-Aging Treatment

The first thing that comes to mind is: Can stem cell therapy cure aging? Well, this book focuses on the probable benefits of stem cell therapy in delaying the aging process. But before that, let us look at what stem cells are.

What are stem cells?

Stem cells are the body's basic materials from which all other cells with specialized roles are generated. Stem cells are unspecialized cells that have not yet decided what form of adult cell they will be. They can self-renew, create two new forms of stem cells, and differentiate to make several types of cells. When a stem cell divides, the two daughter cells that result may be stem cells, a stem cell, and a more developed cell, or both more differentiated cells. The process that governs the balance between both types of divisions to ensure that a suitable amount of stem cells is maintained within a given tissue is not yet fully understood.

The following are the types of stem cells:

1. Embryonic stem cells (ESCs)
2. Adult stem cells (ASCs)
3. Induced pluripotent stem cells (iPSCs)

Anti-aging properties of stem cells

Our present knowledge of human stem cells makes it conceivable to prevent aging and improve health and lifespan. Stem cell treatments can play a vital role in slowing the aging process. Together with anti-aging genes, a stem cell infusion can produce a complex shield that can prevent or reduce the consequences of aging. Increased wear and tear on the body's natural stem cells increases cellular damage and accelerates the natural aging process. Stem cell therapy paired with anti-aging genes can potentially absorb the process of cellular aging.

Regenerative stem cell treatment rejuvenates existing cell types.

Introducing "youthful" human stem cells into the body can renew existing cells, allow the body to age more gracefully, and even reverse some symptoms of the aging process. As we age, our cells get ill and die.

When a cell dies, it generates a cascade of events, leading to inflammation and disease that can limit the human lifetime. There are various methods by which stem cells may be able to prevent aging, including:

1. Regenerating injured tissue: Stem cells can develop into many cell types and can be used to replace damaged tissue, potentially reversing the effects of aging.

2. Enhancing repair mechanisms: Stem cells can promote the creation of growth factors and other signaling molecules that can boost the body's repair processes, helping to retain healthy tissue and postpone the beginning of age-related alterations.

3. Modulating the immune system: Stem cells may have immunomodulatory effects, which could help to maintain a healthy immune system and delay the onset of age-related immune dysfunction.

4. Reducing inflammation: Some research has suggested that stem cells may have anti-inflammatory actions, which could help lessen the persistent low-grade inflammation associated with aging.

5. Protecting against oxidative stress: Stem cells may be able to guard against oxidative stress, which is a process that can lead to cell damage and is thought to play a part in aging.

The advantages of employing stem cell therapy in addressing aging process

- A sensation of vibrancy and regeneration
- Improved capacity for active activities
- Thickening and better quality of hair
- Increased libido
- A decrease in pain
- Increased strength, balance, and general mobility
- Enhanced immunity
- Enhancement of overall life quality
- Immune system modulation

Stem cell anti-aging: how our cells age

Aging is a complex, natural process; the effect of environmental variables, genetics, and ordinary wear and use on the body eventually takes a toll in many ways. It is this effect of life that can cause unavoidable health concerns.

Over time, the cells of the body age as we do, resulting in their incapacity to multiply; they become damaged and die. The decrease in inefficient cell reproduction is what causes our bodies to age.

Anti-aging treatment

Stem cells are a promising possible approach for reversing the outward indications of aging. These particular cells can rebuild damaged tissues and improve general cellular function, which may contribute to a reduction in the appearance of wrinkles and other age-related changes. Some studies have suggested that stem cells may have anti-aging effects on the skin by increasing the creation of collagen, a protein that gives skin its suppleness and strength. While additional research is needed to properly understand the potential of stem cells for anti-aging treatments, the early results are promising and suggest that stem cells may play a crucial role in the development of successful anti-aging medicines in the future.

What are the ten indications of aging?

Some of the most prevalent indicators of aging are:

- Impaired vision
- Impaired hearing
- Loss of strength in muscles
- Loss of bone density
- Decreased immune system function
- Decreased cognitive abilities
- Less efficient metabolism
- Loss of energy
- Hair loss
- Decreased balance and overall mobility

Reversing Aging

Stem cells are a type of cell that can develop into any form of cell in the body. They can divide and duplicate endlessly, making them a viable answer for reversing the aging process. Studies have demonstrated that stem cells can rebuild damaged tissues, reduce inflammation, and improve general cellular function, which may contribute to a reduction in the obvious indications of aging.

Additionally, stem cells can influence the immune system, which may help to improve overall health and well-being as we age. While additional research is needed to properly grasp the potential of stem cells for reversing aging, the early results are promising and imply that stem cells may play a major role in the fight against aging.

So, can stem cells reverse aging?
1. A study published in the journal Aging Cell discovered that bone marrow stem cells can restore the function of aged immune cells and increase the lifespan of mice. The study implies that bone marrow stem cells may have anti-aging effects by lowering inflammation and enhancing immunological function.
2. A study published in the Journal of Aging Research & Clinical Practice reviewed the outcomes of many trials on the use of stem cells for the treatment of age-related disorders. The review found that stem cells can restore damaged tissues, improve organ function, and lower the risk of age-related disorders.

3. A study published in the journal Stem Cells Translational Medicine discovered that stem cells can improve skin health and minimize the appearance of wrinkles in mice. The study implies that stem cells may have anti-aging effects on the skin by increasing the creation of collagen, a protein that gives skin its flexibility and strength.

While these results are intriguing, it's crucial to remember that additional study is needed to properly grasp the potential of stem cells for reversing aging. It's also crucial to highlight that stem cells are not a magic bullet, and their use should be approached with caution and under the advice of a skilled medical professional.

Stem cell treatment for anti-aging

Aging cells can contribute to disease. Thus, if cell aging can be prevented, slowed down, or even reversed, many diseases could be better managed. Stem cells may be able to slow down this process and treat certain age-related disorders.

How do stem cells halt the aging process?

With stem cell therapies, you are renewing the supply of stem cells to allow the body to repair and regenerate all the organs of your body.

Stem cells possess unique elements that aid in anti-aging by helping our bodies rebuild biological tissues, such as:

• Skin

• Joints

• Bones

• Organs

This sophisticated therapy may be able to restore tissue that has been damaged by stress, injury, and environmental causes.

What is stem cell treatment?

During stem cell treatment at DVC Stem (a stem cell clinic based in Grand Cayman), a patient receives roughly 300 million stem cells. These stem cells are taken from umbilical cord samples, all of which undergo comprehensive testing to verify sterility and viability (% of live cells).

DVC Stem then bundles the stem cells and preserves them in a cryogenic condition (colder than 100 degrees below zero). At the moment of intravenous delivery, the cells are thawed to body temperature in a sterile lab and administered over many hours by our highly experienced physicians.

A stem cell transplant tries to replenish the reserve of stem cells practically lost over the last 15–20 years. After such a massive cell replenishment, the body's organs are revitalized and renewed.

Stem cells, those adaptable engineers of life, have emerged as heroes in the fight against aging. Regenerative medicine, the discipline that harnesses the potential of these cells, has promise in not simply delaying the apparent signs of aging but potentially reversing them. Imagine a future where damaged tissues can be rejuvenated, organs can be regenerated, and the deterioration of aging can be held at bay. This is the universe of stem cells and regenerative medicine, a realm that continues to evolve and unfold with each scientific achievement.

Unlocking the Code of Genetic Therapies

BEIJING (Reuters) Scientists in Beijing have created a new gene therapy that can cure some of the symptoms of aging in mice and extend their lifespans, findings that may one day contribute to comparable treatment for people.

The strategy, reported in a publication in the Science Translational Medicine journal earlier this month, involves inactivating a gene called kat7, which the authors identified as a crucial contributor to cellular aging.

Cellular senescence, a state of irreversible growth stop, has emerged as a hallmark and essential cause of organismal aging. It is influenced by both genetic and epigenetic factors. Despite a few previously discovered age-associated genes, the identity and roles of additional genes involved in the control of human cellular aging continue to be understood. Yet, there is a paucity of comprehensive inquiry into the intervention of these genes to treat aging and aging-related disorders.

What is the count of genes in the human genome that contribute to the promotion of aging?

What are the biological mechanisms by which these genes affect aging? Can gene therapy ease individual aging? Recently, experts from the Chinese Academy of Sciences have shed new light on the regulation of aging.

Lately, a collaborative effort between researchers at the Institute of Zoology of the Chinese Academy of Sciences (CAS), Peking University, and the Beijing Institute of Genomics of CAS resulted in the identification of novel human senescence-promoting factors, by employing a comprehensive CRISPR/Cas9 screening system across the genome, the researchers aim to present a fresh therapeutic strategy for addressing both aging and aging-related pathologies

In this paper, the researchers conducted genome-wide CRISPR/Cas9-based screenings in human premature aging stem cells and discovered more than 100 potential senescence-promoting genes. They also tested the efficiency of inactivating each of the top 50 potential genes in promoting cellular rejuvenation using targeted sgRNAs.

Among these, KAT7, which encodes a histone acetyltransferase, was identified as one of the top targets for reducing cellular senescence.

It increases in human mesenchymal progenitor cells during physiological and pathological aging. KAT7 depletion decreased cellular senescence, but KAT7 overexpression promoted cellular senescence. Mechanistically, inhibition of KAT7 lowered histone H3 lysine 14 acetylation, suppressed p15INK4b transcription, and regenerated senescent human stem cells. Cumulative studies have demonstrated that age-associated accumulation of senescent cells and proinflammatory cells in tissues and organs contributes to the genesis and progression of aging as well as aging-related illnesses. Prophylactic ablation of senescent cells mitigates tissue deterioration and extends the health span of mice.

In this investigation, scientists discovered that administering a lentiviral vector containing Cas9/sg-KAT7 through intravenous injection reduced the proportions of senescent cells and proinflammatory cells in the liver, diminished circulatory senescence-associated secretory phenotype (SASP) factors in the serum and extended the health and lifespan of aged mice.

These data imply that gene therapy based on single-factor inactivation may be adequate to enhance mouse lifespan.

The researchers also showed that therapy with the lentiviral vector encoding Cas9/sg-KAT7 or the KAT7 inhibitor WM-3835 relieved human hepatocyte senescence and lowered the expression of SASP genes, suggesting the possibility of implementing these therapies in clinical settings.

Altogether, this study has successfully increased the list of human senescence-promoting genes using the CRISPR/Cas9 genome-wide screen and has proven that gene therapy based on single-factor inactivation can prevent individual aging. This discovery not only increases our understanding of the aging mechanism but also gives us new prospective targets for aging therapies.

Genetic medicines, once the stuff of dreams, are becoming a reality. These medicines have the power to change the instructions coded within our DNA, possibly addressing the core causes of aging.

Imagine a world where genetic medicines can repair broken strands of DNA, reinforce cellular repair systems, and enhance the body's inherent defenses against the passage of time. This realm is on the horizon, with researchers and scientists pioneering medicines that may hold the secrets to an ageless future.

The Symphony of Epigenetics: Rewriting the Story of Aging

Within the genetic script lurks an additional layer of complexity: epigenetics. Epigenetics refers to the modifications to our genes that occur without affecting the underlying DNA sequence. It's a dynamic, responsive layer that is influenced by our lifestyle, surroundings, and experiences.

Epigenetic modification treatment

Other promising ways to treat diseases involve change at the genetic level without affecting the nucleic acid sequences. These procedures affect the expression of genetic information, such as inactivating a disease-causing gene, activating antagonist genes of the disease-causing genes, altering the imbalance in gene expression, or rectifying aberrant chemical alterations.

With advances in the expanded CRISPR/Cas effector technology, tools such as CRISPRa/CRISPRi (directly regulating gene expression), CRISPRoff (initiating DNA methylation), TET3-fused high-fidelity catalytically inactive Cas9 (dCas9) (demethylating methylated DNA), and Cas13-directed methyltransferase (mediating efficient m6A modifications in endogenous RNA transcripts) have been constructed and developed. These instruments enable a broader range of precise epigenetic alterations compared to those facilitated by regulatory noncoding RNAs, such as short hairpin RNA (shRNA) and small interfering RNA (siRNA). Therefore, the operating techniques for epigenetic regulation are leaning toward uniformity. This technique is currently under development and has been largely tested for treating malignant tumors and CRISPR screening in vivo. Recent developments in epigenetics provide a stunning revelation: the possibility to reverse the hallmarks of aging not merely by altering the genetic code but by modifying the "on" and "off" switches that control its expression. Epigenetic changes can mute genes associated with aging and activate those that promote vitality and longevity.

The Frontier of Ageless Alchemy: A Glimpse into Tomorrow

As we explore the world of stem cells, regenerative medicine, genetic medicines, and epigenetics, we stand at the threshold of ageless alchemy. This chapter uncovers the gems of a toolset that defies traditional bounds. It presents us with a symphony of possibilities, a future where the Fountain of Youth isn't a magical spring but a technological miracle within our grasp.

Chapter 4

Turning Back Time: Practical Steps to Ageless Beauty

In the magnificent symphony of life, each note echoes with time, building a melody that dances between the lines inscribed into our skin. But what if we could recreate this symphony, reverse the tempo of aging, and paint a painting of perpetual beauty? In this chapter, we continue on a trip that connects science and art, uncovering practical techniques to not just seem young but to radiate timeless beauty.

A Step-by-Step Guide to Reversing the Clock

Picture a mirror that reflects not just your appearance but also your aspirations, dreams, and the vitality that dwells within. This step-by-step guide is a mirror that uncovers a fresh reflection, one that defies age and celebrates energy. It begins with knowing the science of aging we have examined so far and grows into tangible strategies that enable you to take control of your look.

Unveiling the Artistry of Skincare and Fashion

Skincare is an art, a canvas upon which the brushstrokes of science merge with the hues of self-care. Dive into a skincare routine that is not just about creams and lotions but about caring for your skin from within. Discover makeup techniques that highlight your unique traits, transforming cosmetics into weapons of empowerment rather than masks of hiding.

As we age, we all want to maintain a youthful appearance and slow down the indications of aging. Various revolutionary anti-aging practices might help us obtain a more youthful look. If you're in your 20s or 30s, it's the perfect time to prevent the indications of aging. Take care of your skin while you're young. Many people try to correct the problem when it happens instead of taking care of the problem before it occurs, i.e., fine lines and wrinkles.

Taking care of your skin through a thorough skincare routine and making healthy lifestyle choices can work wonders in preserving a youthful shine.

Here are some key suggestions and habits to safeguard your skin throughout this era of life:

- **Embrace Moisture & Hydration** - Our skin loses moisture and grows drier as we age. Moisturize regularly to retain skin suppleness and decrease the appearance of fine lines and wrinkles. Choose a thick, moisturizing moisturizer suitable for your skin type and apply it routinely in the morning and at night. Look for products containing hyaluronic acid, glycerin, or ceramides, as these efficiently seal in moisture, keeping your skin supple and plump. Also, a wonderful approach to start your day is to apply a moisturizer with a built-in SPF to protect your skin.

- **Sun Protection is Non-Negotiable** - Sun protection becomes even more vital in your 40s and beyond. Exposure to harmful UV rays accelerates the aging process, resulting in the development of fine lines, wrinkles, and dark spots. More significantly, effective sunscreen use can drastically minimize your risk of skin cancer. Make it a habit to integrate a broad-spectrum sunscreen with at least SPF 30 into your daily routine, regardless of the weather.

Eternal beauty is not about halting or reversing time; it's about achieving a state where you both look and feel your very best. Sunscreen isn't just for holidays. SPF should not be weather-dependent but should be part of your regular health and skincare program. Regardless of the weather, be it rainy or sunny, throughout every season, applying sunscreen should be a habitual aspect of your daily routine, like brushing your teeth. Even on days with clouds and overcast skies, damaging rays can permeate the skin.

Daily use of SPF 50 helps protect your skin from dangerous rays that damage and age the skin. To gain UVA protection, check the ingredient list for avobenzone, mexoryl, zinc oxide, or titanium dioxide.

Reapply the sunscreen as indicated on the label. Most people don't put on enough, so be generous when you apply it, and reapply it every one to three hours, depending on the amount of sweating, swimming, or direct sun exposure you get. Nothing is going to work if you don't put on enough and apply it often enough. Don't forget your neck, hands, and arms.

o **Exfoliate Gently** - Regular exfoliation is necessary to eliminate dead skin cells, allowing skincare products to penetrate deeper. However, in your 40s, the skin may become more sensitive, making it vital to exfoliate lightly. Use a moderate exfoliator with substances like alpha hydroxy acids (AHAs) or beta hydroxy acids (BHAs) to encourage skin renewal without irritating. Aim to exfoliate 1-2 times weekly to maintain a smooth and bright complexion.

o **Embrace Retinoids for Skin Renewal** - Retinoids, which come from vitamin A, are famous for their ability to promote collagen formation and improve skin texture. With long-term use, they aid in significantly minimizing the appearance of fine lines and wrinkles while enhancing skin tone and suppleness.

If you just have one anti-aging product in your medicine cabinet, make it a retinoid. Dermatologists promote the strong skincare component (a derivative of vitamin A) for its ability to speed cell renewal. Retinoids reduce fine lines, wrinkles, uneven skin tone, pigmentation, and texture and stimulate collagen formation.

Retinoids flip over skin cells and stimulate collagen formation, which leads to more youthful-looking skin. Are you new to retinoids? The chemical can initially dry your skin or produce additional acne. So, start cautiously by using the retinoid every other day and selecting products with a lesser proportion in your routine. Then, progressively work your way up to utilizing the product every day, or try a higher percentage.

It is vital to contact your dermatologist about the strength and frequency with which to use a retinoid to improve your skin's health and minimize side effects like excessive dryness.

- **Stay Hydrated from the Inside Out** - Proper hydration is crucial for general health and plays a vital role in ensuring your skin stays hydrated and plump. Additionally, go for foods rich in water content, such as fruits and vegetables, to enhance your skin's moisture levels and retain a beautiful glow.

  Antioxidants are your partners - Antioxidants are important partners in the struggle against aging. They neutralize free radicals, unstable chemicals that damage skin cells and cause premature aging.

Include antioxidant-rich skincare products, such as vitamin C serums or creams containing vitamins E and A, to help protect your skin from environmental stresses and promote a more youthful complexion.

o   **Address the eye area with care.** The skin around the eyes is sensitive and reveals signs of aging earlier than in other places. Invest in a quality eye cream formulated to alleviate fine wrinkles, puffiness, and dark circles. Apply it lightly using your ring finger to avoid pulling and limit damage to the sensitive skin.

Applying rose hip oil, olive oil, and coconut oil to your eyelashes and brows will help them grow quicker and appear fuller.

o   **Avoid smoking**

Smoking is terrible news for every part of you. In your skin, it speeds up the breakdown of collagen and constricts blood vessels that transport oxygen and nutrients to your skin. Smokers are more likely to wrinkle early. In time, their nails and fingertips will turn yellow. Day, a former smoker herself, actively advises smokers to quit. The possibility of wrinkles could be the final bit of drive you need. You may need to attempt multiple times to quit for good, but it's more than worth it.

o   **Avoid excessive alcohol intake.**
Having a drink with a buddy or savoring a glass of wine with dinner is great, they say. However, excessive alcohol consumption leads to skin dehydration and the expansion of blood vessels. If you drink too much, you could develop burst blood vessels and rosacea, a skin ailment defined by redness and small pimples.

o   **Serums with Targeted Benefits** - Tailor your skincare routine with serums that treat specific concerns. Serum's rich with chemicals like niacinamide for hyperpigmentation, peptides for firmness, or hyaluronic acid for hydration can work wonders.

o   **Prioritize Quality Sleep** - Adequate sleep is necessary for your body's overall health and crucial to your skin's regeneration process. Aim for 7-9 hours of sleep each night to help your skin to repair and revitalize.

o   **Make healthy lifestyle choices.** Healthy lifestyle choices positively affect your skin. Avoid smoking, restrict alcohol use, and maintain a balanced diet of antioxidants, vitamins, and minerals. Foods like fruits, vegetables, and fatty fish provide critical nutrients for your skin's health.

o   **Stay Active and Manage Stress** - Regular exercise promotes blood circulation, bringing oxygen and nutrients to your skin. Additionally, adopting effective strategies to handle stress, such as meditation, yoga, or spending time in nature, can lessen the detrimental impact of stress on your skin.

o   **Seek a specialist Skincare Consultation:** Visit a dermatologist or skin care specialist for specialized advice and treatments tailored to your skin's specific needs.

As we age, our skin experiences significant changes that require extra attention and care. Nurturing your skin in your 40s and beyond can help preserve a healthy, youthful complexion. Remember, consistency is crucial for nurturing your skin in your 40s and beyond. Be patient, and with the appropriate care, your skin will remain glowing and healthy for years!

Fashion is a story we tell the world about ourselves. In the story of ageless beauty, fashion becomes a means of expression. Explore alternatives that boost your body's strengths and celebrate its originality. It's not about adhering to trends; it's about establishing a style that matches your confidence and vibrancy.

Fashion can play a crucial influence in helping you look and feel younger. Here are some fashion recommendations for anti-aging:

1. Choose flattering hues: Wearing hues that match your skin tone can make a great difference. Hues that match your skin can enhance your appearance, while the wrong hues might make you look washed out.

2. Invest in Quality materials: Quality materials can increase your overall look and comfort. Natural textiles like cotton, silk, and wool are not only comfy but also age nicely.

3. Tailoring is Key: Properly fitted clothing can make you look more put-together and youthful. Well-tailored garments can provide a more streamlined and attractive silhouette.

4. Opt for Classic Styles: Trends come and go, but classic styles tend to remain ageless. A well-fitted jacket, a white button-down shirt, and a little black dress are all examples of classic clothes that may be adaptable and age-appropriate.

5. Embrace Modern Accessories: You don't have to cling to classic, conservative accessories.

Adding contemporary jewelry, luggage, and shoes will offer a youthful edge to your style.

6. Layer Strategically: Layering can give depth and interest to your look. It can also help you adjust to changing weather conditions. However, be wary of over-layering, which can add bulk and make you look older.

7. Balance Comfort and Style: Comfortable clothing doesn't have to mean losing style. Look for clothes that combine both comfort and a trendy appearance.

8. Sun Protection: Protecting your skin from the sun is one of the most effective anti-aging measures. Wear a wide-brimmed hat and sunglasses, and apply sunscreen daily to keep your skin looking youthful.

9. Footwear Matters: Comfortable, supportive shoes may make a world of difference in how you feel and appear. Avoid too high heels that might cause discomfort and back problems.

10. Grooming and Personal Care: Your grooming and personal care routine also play a factor in how youthful you look. Keep your hair well-maintained, pay attention to your skincare, and consider a pleasing haircut.

11. Posture: Good posture can quickly make you look more confident and youthful. Stand up tall and walk with confidence.

12. Experiment, but Stay True to Your Style: While it's fantastic to experiment with your fashion choices, it's crucial to maintain your style. Don't try to look like someone you're not; instead, adjust these guidelines to your preferences.

Remember, fashion is a form of self-expression, and the most essential thing is to feel confident and comfortable in what you wear. These recommendations are not about keeping to rigorous standards but about embracing fashion as a tool to improve your inherent beauty and confidence at any age.

Elevating Confidence and Embracing Evolving Beauty in Anti-Aging Process

Aging is a normal and inevitable aspect of life, and it's a journey that should be embraced with confidence and happiness. As we age, it's crucial to address not just the physical components of anti-aging but also the psychological and emotional parts, particularly when it comes to creating and maintaining good self-esteem.

Confidence and self-assurance play a significant role in how we view our evolving beauty during the anti-aging process. Here's a comprehensive note on raising confidence and accepting and developing attractiveness as we age:

Embrace the Natural Process

Aging is not something to be feared; rather, it's a privilege denied to many. Embracing the natural process of aging is the first step in creating healthy self-esteem as we get older. It's vital to understand that aging is not the enemy but rather the accumulation of life experiences, wisdom, and personal progress. By viewing aging as a natural evolution, you can free yourself from the artificial cultural norms of youth and perfection.

Self-Reflection and Self-Acceptance

Self-reflection is a strong tool for improving self-esteem. As we mature, we should take the time to reflect on our successes, life experiences, and the wisdom we've gathered along the way. Recognize that beauty is not tied to youth; it evolves with time.

Self-acceptance, regardless of age or physical changes, is the foundation of a positive self-image.

Holistic Well-Being

To feel good on the exterior, it's necessary to nurture the inside. A balanced diet, regular exercise, and proper sleep all contribute to feeling better about yourself as you age. These habits not only help preserve physical health but also increase your confidence and self-esteem. Proper self-care sends a powerful statement that you respect yourself and your well-being.

Positive Self-Talk

The way you speak to yourself matters greatly. Negative self-talk can damage self-esteem, while positive affirmations can elevate it. Instead of obsessing over perceived shortcomings or worrying about wrinkles and gray hair, focus on your strengths, your unique talents, and the events that have shaped you. Practice positive self-talk to increase confidence.

Embrace Your Style

As you age, your fashion and style tastes may evolve. Embrace this transition by finding a style that makes you feel comfortable and confident. Rather than pursuing the latest trends, wear attire that improves your self-expression.

Your wardrobe selections should represent your changing personality, and this is a strong method to improve your confidence.

Learn New Skills

Never stop learning. Engaging in new activities or obtaining new abilities not only keeps your mind sharp but also enhances your self-esteem. Whether it is learning a new language, taking up a hobby, or collecting new knowledge, it promotes the concept that you are capable of growth and adaptation.

Surround Yourself with Positive Influences

Your self-esteem is significantly influenced by the individuals you surround yourself with. Seek out friends and loved ones who offer support, encouragement, and positivity. Positive connections can increase your self-esteem and provide a strong support system as you negotiate the aging process.

Seek Professional Guidance

If you discover that your self-esteem and confidence are adversely harmed by aging, consider seeking the help of a therapist or counselor. They can help you address any deeper emotional difficulties associated with aging and provide solutions for creating stronger self-esteem.

In conclusion, embracing evolving beauty in the anti-aging process is not just about skincare and cosmetic operations; it's about cultivating a good self-image and a strong feeling of self-worth. As we age, it's vital to respect our unique path and accept that our beauty evolves with us. Confidence and self-esteem are powerful assets in feeling and looking your best, regardless of age. Celebrate the wisdom and experiences that come with aging, and let them shine through as your most beautiful traits.

Chapter 5

The Ultimate Anti-Aging Diet: Nourishing for Eternal Youth

Beautiful, bright skin starts with how we eat, but these anti-aging foods can also help with more than that.

Our diet is directly related to our skin health and plays a significant part in slowing down age indications. It is always advisable to start early and pack your diet with the best anti-aging nutrients for your skin.

When we pack our diet with vivid foods laden with antioxidants, good fats, water, and critical nutrients, our body will communicate its appreciation through its largest organ: our skin. After all, the skin is frequently the first part of our body to betray internal illness, and there is only so much that lotions, creams, masks, and serums can do before we need to take a deeper look at what is feeding us.

Researchers have also found that eating fruits and veggies is the safest and healthiest strategy to counteract dull complexions and fine wrinkles. Ready to look younger via your meal? Here are the top 40 anti-aging foods to nourish your body for a glow that comes from inside.

Before we dig into the top 40 anti-aging foods that will make you seem younger, let us look at the vital nutrients that keep you youthful.

Essential Nutrients That Keep You Young

Fresh and healthy food offers vitamins, nutrients, and antioxidants that keep your cells alive and prevent any age-related disorders. These nutrients battle the damaging free radicals that damage your skin, therefore lowering the indications of aging dramatically. The necessary nutrients include:

• **Amino Acids:** Stimulate elastin and collagen formation, giving the skin a wrinkle-free and smooth appearance.

• **Carotenoids (Retinol, Beta-Carotene, Vitamin A):** Fight the dangerous free radicals. A study indicated that those with high levels of carotenoids (antioxidants) in Polyphenols: The ingestion of polyphenols protects you from UV damage. They are effective antioxidant and anti-inflammatory agents and have anti-DNA damage effects. Their system had younger-looking skin.

• **Omega-3 Fatty Acids:** They contain anti-inflammatory qualities, and their supplements have been demonstrated to slow down the aging process.

• **Polyphenols:** The ingestion of polyphenols protects you from UV damage. They are powerful antioxidant and anti-inflammatory agents and have anti-DNA damage properties.

• **Vitamin D:** This vitamin protects your skin cells from damage due to UV exposure, inhibits skin infections, and has an anti-aging impact.

• **Selenium:** It increases the antioxidant defenses of your skin, protects the skin cells from UV damage, and has anti-inflammatory benefits.

• **Vitamin C:** It protects your skin against pollution and other environmental effects, stimulates collagen formation, and exhibits antioxidant capabilities.

• **Vitamin E:** It protects your skin from oxidative stress, therefore reducing long-term problems such as wrinkles, edema, erythema, and thickness of the skin.

• **Flavonoids:** They prevent oxidative stress, therefore preventing the indications of aging.

• **Green Tea Polyphenols:** The topical application or eating of green tea polyphenols protects against damage caused by UV radiation and chemical carcinogens. The tea contains anti-inflammatory effects that prevent antioxidant depletion on your skin.

You will find all these anti-aging minerals and vitamins in select food items. Here is the list of the top 40 anti-aging foods for younger-looking skin.

Top 40 Anti-aging Foods That Make You Look Younger

o **Fruits**

1. Avocado

Avocado is one of the anti-aging foods with immense health advantages. It is rich in potassium, vitamins A, C, E, and K, and antioxidants that counteract the effects of aging. Moreover, it is helpful for your general health.

Direction for use:

You may mash avocados and use them as a spread for your toast or simply slice them and add them to your daily salad.

2. Papaya

This delectable superfood is packed with a range of antioxidants, vitamins, and minerals that may aid in enhancing skin suppleness and lessen the appearance of fine lines and wrinkles. These include:

• vitamins A, C, K, and E

• calcium

• potassium

• magnesium

• phosphorus

• B vitamins

The vast spectrum of antioxidants in papaya helps to fight free radical damage and may delay indications of aging. Papaya also contains an enzyme called papain, which provides further anti-aging effects by operating as one of nature's best anti-inflammatory medicines. It's a common ingredient in numerous exfoliating products.

So certainly, eating papaya (or utilizing products containing papain) may help your body shed dead skin cells, leaving you with bright, vivid skin!

Direction for use:

Drizzle fresh lime juice over a huge dish of papaya as part of your breakfast, or prepare a papaya mask at home for your next night!

3. Blueberries

Blueberries contain abundant vitamins A and C, along with an antioxidant known as anthocyanin that combats aging. This is what gives blueberries their rich, gorgeous blue hue.

These potent antioxidants may help protect skin from damage due to the sun, stress, and pollution by modulating the inflammatory response and avoiding collagen loss.

Direction for use:

Throw this delightful, low-sugar fruit into a morning smoothie or fruit bowl, and let it deliver a beautifying punch!

Also, a face pack with a handful of blueberries, yogurt, honey, and olive oil can be produced and used twice a week for good skin.

4. Watermelon

Watermelon not only provides reprieve during hot and humid days, but it also protects your skin from premature aging. This fruit is rich in vitamins C, E, and K, selenium, calcium, manganese, potassium, protein, and carbs.

Direction for use:

There are numerous ways to consume this summer fruit, but you may just slice it or chop it in parts, sprinkle some pepper, and eat.

5. Pomegranates

The ruby red seeds of pomegranate include essential chemicals such as vitamins C, D, E, and K, along with selenium, magnesium, and proteins. These healthful fruits also include a substance called punicalagin, which may aid in retaining collagen in the skin, reducing indications of aging.

All these substances have an anti-aging impact and assist your body in fighting diseases and the indications of aging.

Direction for use:

Add pomegranate to your smoothies and salads for that added crunch, or you can eat it as it is.

Research has also indicated that a chemical called urolithin A, which is formed when pomegranates interact with gut flora, may revitalize mitochondria. It was even observed to reverse muscle aging in rat trials.

6. Strawberries

These juicy red fruits are a powerhouse of critical vitamins. They are filled with phenolic chemicals that have antioxidant and anti-inflammatory properties. They promote cellular metabolism and cell resurrection, avoiding oxidative stress and slowing down the aging process.

Direction for use:

Add strawberries to your salads, smoothies, tarts, and cake toppings.

7. Tomatoes

Tomatoes contain lycopene. This is a non-provitamin A carotenoid that protects your skin from UV damage.

Moreover, the skin of tomatoes has an anti-inflammatory impact on the human skin, and the flavonoids in the fruit slow down aging.

Direction for use:

Tomatoes can be used in your curries, spaghetti, and salads to offer that wonderful zing to your cuisine.

8. Figs

This fruit is filled with polyphenols and flavonoids that give it antioxidant characteristics. Figs inhibit numerous types of oxidative stress, thereby keeping your skin and system healthy.

Direction for use:

Make fig tarts slice them, and add them to your pizza or fruit salad -there are plenty of ways to consume figs.

9. Lemons

Lemons and limes are good sources of vitamin C that help in keeping your skin healthy and radiant. Vitamin C is a vital antioxidant that protects your skin from the impacts of free radicals. They also include flavonoids that are healthy for the skin.

Direction for use:

When life provides you with lemons, you can create lemon juice and lemon tarts, sprinkle them on your salads or barbecues, or just add them to your fresh fruit bowl for an extra zing.

o **Vegetables**

10. Carrots

These crunchy and delicious vegetables are rich providers of beta-carotene, potassium, and antioxidants. They promote weight loss and keep your skin healthy.

Direction for use:

Carrots can be eaten raw, or you can juice it, add it to your stir-fry and salads, and then consume it.

11. Spinach

Spinach is a good source of vitamin A (it contains carotenoids), vitamin C (promotes skin health), folic acid (fosters cell activity), and iron (keeps your tissues robust). It is also rich in antioxidants that help you acquire younger-looking skin.

Direction for use:

Saute spinach leaves with olive oil and a little garlic, or stir-fry it with a bit of low-fat cream cheese.

The simplest way to consume spinach is by adding a handful of leaves to your smoothie and pureeing it.

12. Broccoli

Broccoli is plentiful in vitamins C and K1, potassium, folate, and other minerals. The remarkable antioxidant levels in this vegetable establish it as the ultimate superfood, aiding in the battle against aging indicators.

Direction for use:

Probably the best way to consume broccoli is by steaming it and then adding a bit of salt, olive oil, and vinegar. You have the option to roast it and consume it.

13. Cucumber

It includes 96% water and is rich in antioxidants that minimize oxidative stress in your body. It also contains tannins and flavonoids that prevent the damaging free radicals.

Direction for use:

Sliced cucumbers with a bit of pepper, salt, and lemon are incredibly refreshing on a hot summer day.

14. Red Cabbage

Compared to its green version, red cabbage is higher in lutein, beta-carotene, and antioxidants.

This not only maintains the health of your system but also decelerates the aging process.

Direction for use:

Red cabbage is easy to make. Include raw red cabbage in your salads. You can make pickles with red cabbage or attempt something special like creating potato and cabbage hash.

15. Sweet Potatoes

The inclusion of beta-carotene gives them their orange hue. Sweet potatoes are high in antioxidants and have nearly no fat, carbs, and proteins. They also have anti-inflammatory effects.

Direction for use:

To eat sweet potatoes, you may chop them in chunks and then boil them or just roast unpeeled sweet potato and then have it with a little herb and olive oil.

16. Brussel Sprouts

They are especially high in vitamins C and K (28). While vitamin K is essential for your bone health, vitamin C is an antioxidant that strengthens your immunity and keeps your skin healthy. Brussels sprouts help minimize oxidative stress in your skin cells.

Direction for use:

You may just roast Brussels sprouts with salt and pepper or blanch it, then stir-fry it with onion and garlic. Or simply steam it, add a little lemon juice, pepper, salt, and feta cheese, and delight!

17. Chaga Mushrooms

They are also known as therapeutic mushrooms as they contain high levels of antioxidants. They have anti-inflammatory qualities and prevent cell damage and the impacts of damaging free radicals.

Direction for use:

It's a bit tough for humans to consume raw chaga mushrooms. So, the ideal approach to consume it is by utilizing a chaga mushroom extract (which you can easily buy) and then mixing a few drops with your regular tea or juice.

18. Brinjal

Also known as eggplant or aubergine, this purple vegetable is filled with anthocyanins. These are a sort of flavonoids that destroy dangerous free radicals from your body, keeping your skin youthful.

Direction for use:

Brinjals can be consumed in several ways. Make a dip with them (Baba Ghanoush), roast it, and savor it with a bit of salt, pepper, and chopped onions, or just fry it in a dab of mustard oil.

19. Watercress

The health advantages of watercress don't disappoint! This nutrient-dense moisturizing leafy green is a fantastic source of:

• calcium

• potassium

• manganese

• phosphorus

• vitamins A, C, K, B-1, and B-2 are all included.

Watercress functions as an internal skin disinfectant and enhances the circulation and delivery of minerals to all cells of the body, resulting in better oxygenation of the skin. Loaded with vitamins A and C, the antioxidants in watercress can counteract detrimental free radicals, helping to keep fine lines and wrinkles away.

Direction for use:

Add a handful of this tasty green to your salad today for glowing skin and overall better health.

o **Beverages**

20. Red Wine

This is the latest tool to include in your anti-aging armory. Red wine includes resveratrol, which mimics the benefits that you get with exercise and a low-calorie diet. It assists in regenerating your cells and slows down the aging process. More cause to say cheers!

Direction for use:

A 5-ounce glass a day of this healthful drink is excellent for your health. However, too much of it can be equally hazardous for you.

21. Almond Milk (Fortified)

Almond milk includes a high amount of vitamin E. Just 28 grams of almond milk supplies you with 37% of your daily intake of vitamin E. It protects your skin from the destructive effects of free radicals. When enriched, almond milk also serves as a provider of vitamin D and calcium, similar to dairy milk.

Direction for use:

Almond milk is one of the greatest options for those who want to avoid dairy. Make smoothies or simply drink them without any sugar or added flavors.

22. Green Tea

Green tea includes polyphenols that increase the formation of keratinocytes, thereby slowing down the aging process of your skin. Moreover, it minimizes the extracellular matrix damage on your skin, thereby minimizing wrinkles.

Direction for use:

Early morning is the optimum time to drink green tea. However, make sure you are not eating green tea more than thrice a day.

Also, mix a spoonful of green tea powder, honey, and milk and use as a scrub. It has strong exfoliating capabilities and can be used twice a week.

o **Herbs & Spices**

23. Parsley

Parsley is not just for garnishing your cuisine, but it also provides a storehouse of vitamins A, C, K, B1, and B3. It is rich in flavonoids, especially luteolin, which protects against oxidative cell damage, keeping your skin bright and healthy.

Direction for use:

Drizzle it in your salad bowl, toss a handful of this herb in your spaghetti, or just add it to your smoothie - parsley may be ingested in different ways.

24. Turmeric

This therapeutic spice is the answer to many health difficulties. And it also has anti-aging qualities. Turmeric includes curcumin, which helps slow down oxidative damage and low-grade inflammation that leads to aging. Both eating and topical application of turmeric are excellent for your skin.

Direction for use:

Turmeric is commonly utilized in Indian cuisines. A Pinch of turmeric in your daily fries, veggies, and a glass of milk is incredibly nutritious.

25. Garlic

A study demonstrates that garlic contains antioxidant, antimicrobial, and detoxifying characteristics that have youth-preserving and anti-aging effects on your skin.

Direction for use:

The ideal method to take garlic is raw (cut it and gulp it with your favorite drink). However, garlic offers a strong and spicy flavor to your roasts and stir-fries.

26. Saffron

This fragrant plant suppresses the action of tyrosinase and lowers melanogenesis (a process via which melanin is formed). This has an anti-aging effect. Moreover, it includes phenolic components such as monoterpenoids, kaempferol, and quercetin that prevent melanogenesis.

Direction for use:

The ideal approach to take saffron is by soaking a few strands in milk and then sipping that saffron milk.

o Other Food Substances

27. Extra Virgin Olive Oil

Extra virgin olive oil includes oleic acid that lowers the effect of C-reactive protein. C-reactive protein is associated with age-related problems. It also inhibits the cell renewal process in your body. By minimizing its effect, olive oil helps you stay young. Extra virgin olive oil stands out as one of the healthiest oils on the planet. It's rich in healthful fats and antioxidants that help reduce inflammation and oxidative damage produced by an imbalance of free radicals in the body.

A diet rich in olive oil has been related to a lower risk of chronic diseases, including:

• heart disease

• type 2 diabetes

• metabolic syndrome

• certain forms of cancer

In particular, monounsaturated fats (MUFAs) make up around 73% of olive oil. Some studies have suggested that a diet rich in MUFAs may help decrease skin aging thanks to the powerful anti-inflammatory effects of these healthy fats.

Extra virgin olive oil is also strong in antioxidants, such as tocopherols and beta carotene, as well as phenolic compounds that also have anti-inflammatory qualities.

For example, one 2012 study indicated that persons who followed a diet rich in MUFAs from olive oil had a decreased risk of severe skin aging.

The authors suggested that the anti-inflammatory effects of both MUFAs and antioxidants contained in olive oil were most likely responsible for this impact.

Ideally, pick cold-pressed extra virgin olive oil because it's stronger in antioxidants and less processed than oils that are extracted using other ways. Consider incorporating it into a salad or as s dipping sauce.

Direction for use:

Mix the olive oil in your salad dressing, use it in the marinades and sauces, or just use it as dips instead of mayo or butter.

28. Salmon

Astaxanthin is the chemical that gives salmon its scarlet hue. It not only inhibits inflammation but also minimizes oxidative stress, therefore slowing down the indications of aging. Furthermore, salmon contains abundant selenium and is high in omega-3 fatty acids.

Research has revealed that omega-3 fatty acids are linked to a strong skin barrier and may help minimize inflammation that damages the skin.

In one study, participants with sun-damaged skin consumed a mixture of astaxanthin and collagen for 12 weeks.

As a result, individuals noticed considerable increases in skin elasticity and moisture.

However, while these results seem encouraging, it's unknown if the effects were attributable to astaxanthin, collagen, or both.

Salmon and other fatty fish are high in protein, which is crucial to eat so your body can build collagen and elastin. These two chemicals are responsible for the skin's strength, plumpness, and suppleness. Eating protein also helps wound healing.

Finally, fish is high in selenium. This mineral and antioxidant play a role in DNA synthesis and repair and may help decrease and prevent skin damage from UV exposure. Having proper amounts in the body may lessen the severity of skin illnesses like psoriasis.

Direction for use:

You can have salmon grilled or roasted or broil it with seasonings and butter.

29. Collagen Protein

Collagen is the most crucial element that helps you stay healthy and young. Marine collagen peptides protect your skin by boosting the antioxidant levels in your body. It also assists in mending and rebuilding your skin. Collagen protein is typically found in foods such as fish, vegetables, citrus fruits, garlic, berries, etc.

Direction for use:

Simply add food items rich in collagen protein to your diet, or you can even purchase collagen protein supplements in the market.

30. Dark Chocolate or Cocoa

Dark chocolate is a high source of polyphenols, which work as antioxidants in the body.

In particular, it includes flavonols, which are associated with several health advantages, such as a lower risk of:

• heart disease

• type 2 diabetes

• cognitive deterioration

Additionally, it's claimed that a diet rich in flavanols and other antioxidants can help protect the skin from solar damage and assist in reducing skin aging.

A study indicated that ingesting dark chocolate reduces wrinkles and preserves skin suppleness and hydration levels. The flavanols contained in dark chocolate reduce the damage caused by UV radiation.

In one high-quality 24-week trial, participants who ingested a flavanol-rich cocoa beverage saw significant improvements in skin elasticity and face wrinkles compared with those in the control group.

While these results are promising, other research has not discovered that dark chocolate delivers benefits for skin look or aging.

Keep in mind that the greater the cocoa content, the greater the flavanol content. Therefore, if you wish to add dark chocolate to your diet, choose a variety with at least 70% cocoa solids and low added sugar.

Direction for use:

Use dark chocolate to adorn your pastries and morning bowl of cereals and oatmeal. If the bitterness isn't a concern for you, consume it in its current state.

31. Beans

Be it soybeans, black beans, or any other variety of beans – they are gifted with anti-aging effects. Beans (particularly black beans) contain anthocyanins and isoflavones. These substances prevent skin aging and damage caused by UV radiation, inflammation, and ROS (Reactive Oxygen Species).

Direction for use:

Add it to the hummus to give it a fun twist, cook black beans with quinoa, or prepare a healthy veggie and bean soup - you can consume beans in any way you choose.

32. Nuts

High amounts of inflammation speed up the aging process. Many nuts (particularly almonds) are a wonderful source of vitamin E (Tocopherol), which may help repair skin tissue, keep skin moisture, and protect skin from damaging UV radiation. Walnuts even include anti-inflammatory omega-3 fatty acids that may help:

• strengthen skin cell membranes

• protect against sun damage

• enhance the radiance of the skin by preserving its natural oil barrier.

Direction for use:

Sprinkle a combination of nuts on top of your salads, or consume a handful as a snack. Don't remove the skin, either, as studies suggest that 50 percent or more of the antioxidants are lost without the skin.

33. Maca

Maca root provides enormous health advantages. A study also demonstrated that when applied to the skin, maca extracts reduce skin damage induced by UV exposure. They include polyphenol antioxidants that keep your skin healthy.

Direction for use:

If you have maca powder, you can add a teaspoon to your morning coffee or put some in your smoothie.

34. Clarified Butter (Ghee)

Ghee is filled with vitamins A, C, D, E, and K. It contains alpha-tocopherol that protects your skin from harm and keeps it youthful.

Direction for use:

Ghee is commonly utilized in Indian cooking. You may use ghee for sauteing, spread it on your baked delicacies instead of butter, or simply use it instead of oil for cooking.

35. Yogurt

This ranks among the widely consumed fermented dairy products. It is rich in gut-friendly microorganisms that act as probiotics. A study claims that probiotics slow down both intrinsic and extrinsic aging and keep your skin shining.

Direction for use:

You can consume plain yogurt or blitz it a bit with your favorite fruit to add some flavor. Yogurt can be used as a dip or as a salad dressing in place of mayonnaise.

36. Oatmeal

Oatmeal includes avenanthramide. This chemical is only found in oats and is a potent antioxidant. It possesses anti-inflammatory and antioxidant qualities that help in slowing down aging.

Direction for use:

Start your day with a bowl of oats and warm milk, or mix it with a touch of yogurt, dried fruits, and sliced fresh fruits and transform it into delectable muesli.

37. Sesame Seeds

Sesame seeds contain sesamin. This is a form of lignan (phytoestrogens) that has anti-aging benefits on the skin.

Direction for use:

Chewing raw sesame seeds in the morning is helpful for health. You can consume sesame seed oil. And if you have a sweet tooth, then roast sesame seeds, put them with jaggery, and roll them into little balls.

38. Flax Seeds

Flax Seeds offer amazing health advantages.

They include lignans, which are a type of polyphenol that has antioxidant benefits and may lessen your risk of getting a chronic disease, such as heart disease and breast cancer.

They are also a significant source of an omega-3 fatty acid called alpha-linolenic acid (ALA). Consuming a diet high in omega-3 fats helps support a healthy skin membrane by helping your skin stay moisturized and plump.

In good-quality research from 2009 and 2011, women who consumed flax seeds or flax oil for 12 weeks exhibited enhanced hydration and smoother skin. However, fresh study is needed.

39. Red Bell Pepper

Red bell peppers are filled with antioxidants, which reign supreme when it comes to anti-aging. In addition to their high level of vitamin C— which is helpful for collagen formation — red bell peppers include potent antioxidants called carotenoids.

Carotenoids are plant pigments responsible for the brilliant red, yellow, and orange colors you find in many fruits and vegetables. They offer a variety of anti-inflammatory effects and may help protect skin from sun damage, pollution, and environmental pollutants.

Direction for use:

Slice bell peppers and dip them in hummus as a snack, throw them into a raw salad or boil them up in a stir-fry.

40. Grapefruit

Another fantastic anti-aging food is grapefruit. For years, grapefruit has been widely employed in the area of skincare treatment. Grapefruit is believed to include chemicals that can aid dead skin cells metabolize, therefore making the skin smooth and hydrated.

In conclusion, the foods you eat can play a role in the health of your skin, especially in how your skin changes as you get older.

For instance, diets that are abundant in protein, healthy fats, and antioxidants are connected to the biggest skin advantages.

Along with eating a nutritious diet full of whole, plant-based foods, consider preserving your skin with additional habits, such as wearing sunscreen, avoiding smoking, remaining physically active, and using suitable skin care products.

Nutrition's Role in the Aging Process

Introduction: Aging is a normal and inevitable process that affects every living entity, including humans. While genetics have a key part in determining the rate of aging, current research has indicated that diet plays a crucial role in regulating the aging process. The foods we consume have a dramatic impact on our overall health and can either accelerate or decelerate the aging process. This essay digs into the connection between nutrition and aging, illustrating the different ways in which our dietary choices might affect how we age.

I. **Cellular Aging and Oxidative Stress:**

A. Oxidative Stress and Free Radicals:

1. As we age, our bodies collect damage caused by free radicals, which are unstable chemicals formed during regular cellular activities.

2. Antioxidants, found in numerous foods, can help neutralize free radicals and minimize oxidative stress.

B. Key Nutrients:

1. Vitamins C and E, together with minerals like selenium and zinc, operate as antioxidants, protecting cells from oxidative damage.

2. Consuming foods high in these nutrients can lead to healthier cells and slower aging.

II. **Inflammation and Aging:**

 A. Chronic Inflammation:

1. Low-grade, chronic inflammation is associated with several age-related diseases, such as cardiovascular disease, arthritis, and neurological disorders.

2. Certain meals can either induce or diminish inflammation in the body.

B. **Anti-Inflammatory Foods:**

1. Omega-3 fatty acids found in fish, flaxseeds, and walnuts have anti-inflammatory qualities.

2. A diet rich in fruits, vegetables, and whole grains is connected with reduced levels of inflammation and healthy aging.

III. **Maintaining Muscle Mass and Strength:**

 A. Sarcopenia:

1. Sarcopenia is the age-related loss of muscular mass and strength.

2. Adequate protein consumption, particularly from lean sources, can assist counteract muscle loss.

B. **Protein and Amino Acids:**

1. Protein offers vital amino acids needed for muscle upkeep and repair.

2. Older adults should consume sufficient protein to sustain muscle health.

IV. **Bone Health:**

A. **Osteoporosis:**

1. Osteoporosis, characterized by weakening and brittle bones, is a prevalent condition in aging.

2. Calcium and vitamin D are vital for sustaining bone health.

B. **Nutrients for Bone Health:**

1. Calcium-rich diets like dairy products and fortified plant-based alternatives are needed.

2. Vitamin D, which can be gained from sun exposure and some foods, aids in calcium absorption.

V. **Cognitive Function:**

A. **Neurodegeneration:**

1. Aging is related to cognitive impairment and an increased risk of neurological disorders like Alzheimer's.

2. Certain nutrients improve brain health and cognitive performance.

B. Brain-Boosting Nutrients:

1. Omega-3 fatty acids, present in fatty fish, improve brain function and may lessen the incidence of cognitive decline.

2. Antioxidant-rich diets, including berries, dark leafy greens, and nuts, are associated with higher cognitive function.

Conclusion: Nutrition plays a critical role in the aging process, regulating cellular aging, inflammation, muscle and bone health, and cognitive function. By making appropriate food choices, individuals can promote healthier aging, minimize the risk of age-related disorders, and enhance their overall quality of life. It is crucial to have a balanced diet that contains a variety of nutrient-rich foods to support healthy aging and lessen the harmful impacts of the aging process. Additionally, talking with a healthcare practitioner or registered dietitian can provide specific advice on nutrition for healthy aging.

Crafting Your Personal Ageless Menu: Customizable Meal Plans

This chapter covers not merely theories, but real techniques for designing your timeless menu. Meal plans adapted to individual needs and interests become your brushes, allowing you to explore a palette of flavors, textures, and colors that boost your vitality.

Ageless Mediterranean Dieting with 14-Day Meal Plans

What is The Mediterranean Diet?

The Mediterranean diet is primarily plant-based. Here, People would consume whatever they had growing in their gardens, along with some dairy and olive oil.

The Mediterranean diet is based on the traditional foods of nations bordering the Mediterranean Sea, notably France, Spain, Greece, and Italy.

Some study has revealed that persons living in these places tend to be healthier and have a decreased risk of several chronic illnesses.

The Mediterranean diet often encourages people to:

• **consume more:**

o fruits

o vegetables

o whole grains

o legumes

nuts and seeds

heart-healthy fats

• **consume less:**

processed foods

added sugars

refined grains

• **limit** alcohol consumption

Research has revealed that the Mediterranean diet can:

• promote weight reduction

• help reduce heart attacks, strokes, and type 2 diabetes

• reduce the risk of premature death

For this reason, the Mediterranean diet is a viable alternative for those wishing to improve their health and guard against chronic disease.

Tips for Creating Your Mediterranean Diet Plan

The good news is that because this is a style of eating instead of a set of rigorous rules, you can tailor this method to meet your likes and dislikes.

There's no strict adherence or risk of veering off course and experiencing a sense of failure. "Even within the Mediterranean diet, there are what we call 'special occasion days' where you may eat more or eat foods that perhaps are not very healthy, but that is part of the lifestyle," Paravantes-Hargitt explains. "Food is to be enjoyed, and the Mediterranean diet promotes a healthy relationship with food. 'Cheating' is part of the Mediterranean diet. You just proceed the next day as if nothing happened."

Still, here are five key ideas to get you started:
1. **Eat more legumes.**
 Not only are they a basic that you're probably not eating enough of anyhow, but they're budget-friendly and offer several nutritional benefits, Paravantes-Hargitt, such as being high in fiber and protein, low in fat, and a source of B vitamins, iron, and antioxidants. These encompass dry peas, various beans, lentils, and chickpeas, such as those found in hummus.
2. **Don't overuse booze:**
One widespread mistake is that people following the Mediterranean diet drink a lot of red wine.

In the Mediterranean diet, wine is typically consumed moderately and always accompanies meals. Normally, a small quantity of about 3 to 4 ounces is enjoyed alongside the meal.

3. **Make meat a side**:
Traditionally, people ate meat only for exceptional occasions, such as a Sunday supper, and even then, in tiny portions. Try to add more vegetarian-based mains, such as ones centered around beans, tofu, or seitan, into your day. A solid beginning point is to adopt a vegetarian diet for one day each week. When you do eat meat, focus on selections like skinless chicken and save red meat for once a week or twice a month.

4. **Eat fewer sweets**: Just like meat, make desserts a special occasion dish. That doesn't mean sugar is out— have a bit in your coffee if you'd like, for instance, however, daily, the sugar intake is minimal.

5. Cook using olive oil:

Choose extra-virgin olive oil as your cooking oil. While overdoing it with this oil can contribute to weight gain (it is a fat after all, so the calories can mount up quickly), it's rich in heart-healthy polyunsaturated and monounsaturated fat, so you can feel good about keeping a bottle ready in the kitchen. You may also use it in cold applications to make salad dressing or to sprinkle on cooked veggies or side dishes.

A Complete Mediterranean Food Diet List

Consider these recommendations for including and excluding specific foods when transforming your meals into a Mediterranean-style diet:

Protein

Abundantly Eat:

- Beans
- Lentils
- Chickpeas
- Tofu
- Tempeh
- Seitan

Occasionally Eat:

- Chicken
- Fish
- Seafood
- Eggs

Rarely Eat or Avoid:

- Red meat (beef and pork)
- Cured meats (bacon, sausage, and salami)
- Processed meat items (chicken nuggets)

Oil and Fat

Abundantly Eat:

- Extra-virgin olive oil
- Avocados and avocado oil
- Olives

Occasionally Eat:

- Canola oil

Rarely Eat or Avoid:

- Trans fats
- Margarine
- Butter

Fruits and Veggies

Abundantly Eat:

• Vegetables with low starch content (such as bell peppers, zucchini, eggplant, artichokes, and dark greens)

• Vegetables with higher starch content (sweet potatoes, root vegetables and potatoes)

• Various fruits (apricots, peaches, blueberries, cherries, strawberries, raspberries, and blackberries)

Occasionally Eat:

• There are no off-limits fruits or veggies.

Rarely Eat or Avoid:

• No fruits or veggies are off-limits.

Nuts and Seeds

Abundantly Eat:

• While they can be part of every day, eat them in moderation.

Occasionally Eat:

• Almonds

• Pistachios

• Hazelnuts

• Walnuts

• Cashews (and all other unsweetened nuts)

Rarely Eat or Avoid:

• Sweetened trail mixes

• Sweetened nut butter

• Sugar-coated nuts

Grains

Abundantly Eat:

• Choose whole-grain bread with whole-wheat flour listed as the primary ingredient.

• Opt for whole grains such as bulgur wheat, farro, barley, and quinoa)

• Oatmeal (steel-cut or old-fashioned)

Occasionally Eat:

• Pasta (select whole-wheat pasta whenever possible)

• Couscous

• Whole-grain crackers

• Polenta

• All-bran cereals

Rarely Eat or Avoid:

• Frozen waffles and pancakes

• Sugar-sweetened cereals

• Crackers and other snack foods

Diary

Abundantly Eat:

- These are ingested in moderation.

Occasionally Eat:

- Plain Greek yogurt
- Plain ricotta and cottage cheese
- Milk
- Brie, feta, or goat cheese (plus other cheeses that you prefer)

Rarely Eat or Avoid:

- Ice cream
- Sweetened yogurt
- Processed cheese

Sweeteners

Abundantly Eat:

- These are ingested in moderation.

Occasionally Eat:

- Honey
- A modest amount of added sugar (in coffee or tea, for example)

Rarely Eat or Avoid:

- White sugar

Condiments and Sauces

Abundantly Eat:

- Tomato sauce (no sugar added)
- Pesto
- Balsamic vinegar

Occasionally Eat:

- Aioli
- Tahini
- Tzatziki

Rarely Eat or Avoid:

- Barbecue sauce
- Ketchup
- Teriyaki sauce

Drinks

Abundantly Take:

- Water
- Coffee
- Tea

Occasionally Take:

- Red wine or other alcohol

Rarely take or avoid:

• Soda

• Fruit juice

• Bottled sweetened coffee

Herbs & Spices

Abundantly Eat:

• All dried herbs and spices

• All fresh herbs

• Garlic

Occasionally Eat:

• Salting meals to taste

Rarely Eat or Avoid:

• There's no reason to ban these in your foods.

Effective 14-Day Mediterranean Diet Eating Plan for Anti-Aging

Day 1:

Meal	Food Substances	Snack
Breakfast	Coffee, or tea with a bowl of oatmeal topped with berries	Handful of Almonds or Walnuts
Lunch	Half of a turkey sandwich made with whole-grain bread and a cup of lentil soup	Sliced carrot, bell pepper, and cucumbers dipped in hummus.
Dinner	Veggie and white bean stew	

Day 2:

Meal	Food Substances	Snack
Breakfast	Coffee or tea with plain Greek yogurt topped with a sprinkle of honey and walnuts	Roasted chickpeas
Lunch	Leftover veggie and bean stew from yesterday's meal	A peach (or apple, depending on the season)
Dinner	Grilled chicken accompanied by pita bread and tzatziki, a yogurt-based sauce	

Day 3:

Meal	Food Substances	Snack
Breakfast	Smoothie created with the milk of your choice, fruit, and nut butter	¼ avocado mashed with lemon juice and salt on top of whole grain crackers
Lunch	Three-bean soup topped with a dab of pesto and served with a whole grain bun	Package of olives and fresh veggies.
Dinner	Salmon with farro and grilled zucchini and eggplant	

Day 4:

Meal	Food Substances	Snack
Breakfast	Coffee or tea and toasted whole-grain bread, sliced cheese, and strawberries	Pistachios
Lunch	Lentil-based salad with feta, roasted red peppers, sun-dried tomatoes, and olives	Greek yogurt with fresh fruit
Dinner	Grilled shrimp accompanied by sautéed kale and polenta.	

Day 5:

Meal	Food Substances	Snack
Breakfast	Coffee or tea and a breakfast bowl of leftover farro (from dinner on day 3) topped with a poached egg and a couple slices of avocado	Dried apricots and walnuts
Lunch	Quinoa, bean, and veggie salad served with a slice of whole-grain bread	Whole-grain crackers, and black bean dip.
Dinner	Skewers of marinated and grilled chicken, accompanied by bulgur wheat and a salad of cucumber and red onion.	

Day 6:

Meal	Food Substances	Snack
Breakfast	Coffee or tea and smoked salmon, capers, and tomato slices	In-season fruit (such as a peach or two apricots in summer, or a pear in winter)
Lunch	Mediterranean bean salad and whole-grain crackers	A piece of cheese with olives.
Dinner	Moroccan lamb stew with couscous	

Day 7:

Meal	Food Substances	Snack
Breakfast	Coffee or tea and Greek yogurt with sunflower nuts and raspberries	Sliced orange and pistachios
Lunch	A piece of whole-grain bread with sliced tomatoes, cheese, and olives	Packaged flavored lupini beans
Dinner	Red lentil and vegetable stew	

Day 8:

Meal	Food Substances	Snack
Breakfast	Coffee or tea and two eggs with sautéed greens (spinach or kale), with an orange	Roasted chickpeas
Lunch	Leftover lamb stew from dinner on day 6	Mixed nuts with a chunk of dark chocolate
Dinner	White fish baked in the oven, served with roasted potatoes and zucchini.	

Day 9:

Meal	Food Substances	Snack
Breakfast	Smoothie made with the milk of your choice, frozen cherries, banana, and cocoa powder	Mini peppers filled with hummus
Lunch	Tuna salad cooked with olive oil, dried herbs, olives, and sun-dried tomatoes served over a bed of spinach with mixed veggies and whole-grain crackers	A slice of cheese with a slice of fruit
Dinner	Hearty Tuscan white bean soup with whole-grain bread.	

Day 10:

Meal	Food Substances	Snack
Breakfast	Coffee or tea and a bowl of oats topped with raisins and crumbled walnuts add a drizzle of honey if desired	Greek yogurt, and a piece of fruit
Lunch	Leftover Tuscan white bean soup from dinner on day 9	Hummus with sliced raw veggies like red peppers, celery, and cucumber
Dinner	Garlic lemon chicken thighs paired with asparagus and Israeli couscous.	

Day 11:

Meal	Food Substances	Snack
Breakfast	Coffee or tea with a slice of vegetable frittata with avocado	Apples with nut butter
Lunch	Prepared dolmas (search for these packed grape leaves in the prepared food area at various shops) with hummus and pita	Greek yogurt dip with sliced veggies.
Dinner	A stew of seafood, including shrimp and white fish, in a tomato-based broth.	

Day 12:

Meal	Food Substances	Snack
Breakfast	Coffee or tea and a small bowl of ricotta topped with fruits (berries, peaches, or fresh apricots) with a drizzle of honey	a handful of gently salted nuts (hazelnuts, pistachios, almonds, or a mix)
Lunch	Greek pasta salad (whole-grain pasta with red onion, tomato, Kalamata olives, and feta) served on a bed of romaine	Fruit salad.
Dinner	Remaining seafood stew from the meal on the eleventh day.	

Day 13:

Meal	Food Substances	Snack
Breakfast	Coffee or tea and oats with nut butter and blueberries	Container of Greek yogurt
Lunch	Salmon salad sandwich with a cup of bean-based soup	Smashed avocado on whole-grain crackers
Dinner	Shakshuka (baked eggs in tomato sauce) topped with feta and served over polenta.	

Day 14:

Meal	Food Substances	Snack
Breakfast	Coffee or tea and toasted whole-grain bread topped with ricotta and sliced fruit	Dried cranberries and mixed nuts
Lunch	Quinoa bowl with roasted sweet potatoes, goat cheese, and walnuts	Olives and a couple of pita chips dipped in hummus.
Dinner	Pasta with artichokes and cannellini beans, topped with breadcrumbs and Parmesan cheese.	

Foods to Limit: Junk foods: fast food and potato chips

• **Processed carbohydrates:** pasta, white bread, crackers, flour tortillas, and biscuits

• **Deep-Fried foods:** donuts, French fries, and fried meats

• **Beverages with added sugars:** tea with added sugar, soda, and sports drinks

• **Processed meats:** bacon, canned beef, salami, and sausages

• **Trans fats:** vegetable oil and margarine.

Chapter 6

Sculpting Timeless Bodies: Exercise for the Ages

Exercise can help fight aging by allowing your body to react better to the aging process or create adjustments at the cellular level. Turning back the clock is not only about wrinkles and fine lines. It is about staying fit—not simply looking at it—and keeping your body moving.

We all know that exercise helps to strengthen the strength of the body, provides a boost to muscle mass, and optimizes our health. But it is more exciting to know that exercising reverses the aging process.

Let us begin!

Before anything else, you need to see a doctor before commencing your training quest.

When individuals commence their fitness journey, it becomes crucial to evaluate their physical conditions, because, while there is almost no absolute contraindication to exercise, certain medical or physical issues may demand some adaptations to an exercise plan.

Your physician may wish to make some alterations to your exercise plan. For examples:

• For people with **osteoporosis**, impact activity (with caution) and weight training are crucial because these types of exercise can assist in growing bone mass and halt deterioration.

• For individuals with **arthritis,** impact exercise can be unpleasant to the joints; thus, physicians often recommend low-impact cardiovascular exercises, such as swimming or biking.

• Patients with uncontrolled **high blood pressure** (greater than 180/110 mmHg) should avoid strenuous weightlifting until they've received approval from their doctor.

After gaining the go-ahead from your doctor, it's time to begin: It's ride. It's also smart to start slowly.

The idea is to create a habit and be able to progressively increase your activity over time. If you want to start with lifting weights, then start with weights that you can accomplish 10–12 repetitions of in one set. You wouldn't want to experience such intense soreness after the initial activity that it hinders your ability to move for an entire week.

Take some time to recover!

Fitness recovery is one component of a workout you should take into mind.

Exercising is only part of the battle; it is vital to take adequate care of your body before and after training. That includes being hydrated and nourishing your body with nutritious food. It also includes stretching before and after your workout to help keep your muscles happy and prevent damage.

Fitness recovery doesn't have to be complicated. Find a method that works for you and utilize it often, whether you want:

o Foam rolling

o Massage

o Compression, heat or cold therapy

These should all be complements to mobility work, healthy nutrition, and water.

Don't forget to warm up, either, because launching into your workout without preparing your muscles and joints might lead to damage.

The Anti-Aging Effects of Exercise

The aging process is inherent and leads to alterations in both our physical and mental aspects. While we cannot halt the passage of time, we believe it may actively influence how we age. Regular exercise has emerged as a potent strategy for promoting good aging, giving a plethora of advantages that can promote longevity, vitality, and overall well-being. The benefits of exercise for aging include:

- Physical **health and vitality:**

Regular exercise has a significant role in sustaining physical health and vitality as we age. It helps prevent or manage chronic disorders such as heart disease, osteoporosis, diabetes, and arthritis. Exercise increases cardiovascular fitness, strengthens bones and muscles, and boosts flexibility and balance, reducing the risk of falls and injuries. By keeping the body healthy and functional, exercise allows individuals to maintain independence and an active lifestyle far into their senior years.

- Strengthening **Muscles and Bones:**

As we age, muscle mass and bone density naturally drop.

However, partaking in frequent resistance training exercises, such as weightlifting or bodyweight workouts, can slow down this process. Strength training not only helps grow and maintain muscle mass, but it also strengthens bones, reducing the risk of osteoporosis and fractures. By keeping our muscles and bones strong, we boost our general physical function and independence, promoting a longer and more active life.

- Cognitive **Function and Mental Well-Being:**
Engaging in physical activity benefits not just the body but also contributes to the well-being of the soul. Studies have indicated that physical activity increases cognitive function, memory, and overall mental well-being. Regular exercise boosts blood flow to the brain, encourages the creation of new neurons, and enhances neuroplasticity. It can also lessen the risk of age-related cognitive decline, including illnesses like Alzheimer's disease. Additionally, exercise releases endorphins, boosting a pleasant mood, lowering stress, and battling symptoms of despair and anxiety.

- Enhanced **Quality of Sleep:**
Aging typically poses obstacles to receiving quality sleep.

Regular exercise can help resolve sleep disorders by providing a deeper, more restful sleep. Engaging in physical exercise during the day helps regulate circadian rhythms, promotes the production of sleep-inducing hormones, and minimizes the occurrence of sleep problems. Improved sleep quality leads to greater overall health, increased energy levels, and a sharper intellect.

- **Social Connections and Emotional Well-Being:** Maintaining social relationships and emotional well-being are key parts of good aging. Exercise provides possibilities for social involvement, whether through group fitness programs, walking clubs, or team sports. Participating in these activities provides a sense of belonging, combats loneliness, and promotes a good attitude toward life. Regular exercise also enhances self-esteem, body image, and self-confidence, leading to a positive sense of self as individuals negotiate the aging process.

  - Enhanced **mobility:** Exercise is a crucial factor in increased flexibility, posture, and mobility.
  - Prevents **falls:** Falls are a serious concern when people lose flexibility, strength, and coordination.
  -

- Other risk factors could potentially include disease or incapacity. Exercise can minimize the risk of falls, injuries, and subsequent hospital stays.
- Improves **bone density:** Many elderly people suffer from a condition called osteoporosis, when bones weaken and become more susceptible to fractures. Performing regular resistance training is proven to maintain bone strength in older adults.
- Forms **a cornerstone habit:** Exercise is a habit that has been demonstrated by behavioral scientists to support other useful routines, such as good eating and social contact. Physical activity can, therefore, have a host of good knock-on consequences.
- **It's fun!** Why do youngsters play games? They don't consider the exercise advantages but rather perceive movement as its own reward. Although you might find it hard to return to exercise after a long break, you'll soon love the development as your fitness and mobility levels improve.

Aging gracefully and retaining a high quality of life is within grasp via the power of exercise.

By adding regular physical activity into everyday routines, individuals can improve physical health, retain cognitive function, boost sleep quality, create social relationships, and cultivate emotional well-being. Embracing exercise as a lifelong habit allows us to embrace the process of aging with vitality, joy, and a hopeful outlook.

Five Exercises You Should Do When You Are Over 30
Many think of exercise as the panacea for all of their health woes—even those related to the aging process. Of course, no amount of physical exercise can stop us from getting older, but there's plenty of evidence that indicates that physical activity can extend life expectancy by minimizing the onset and progression of chronic diseases—something many persons start thinking about once they approach 40.
Desire to achieve the peak physical fitness of your life? Follow the workout routines below to help you drop pounds, firm up, and transform your entire body, whether you're in your 40s, 50s, or beyond.

There comes a point in your life when you realize you're no longer invincible. Believe it or not, the body starts to degrade after approximately 30 years, and that decline gets more aggressive every year. The good news: Exercise not only helps you feel (and look!) better, but it can also decrease that decline, helping you stave off several common health concerns.

Below are ten (10) workouts you should start practicing every week once you're in your 40s to stay healthy, happy, and looking as beautiful as you feel.

1. Cardiovascular Workouts (3 to 4 times a week)

Hint: This helps to prevent heart-related problems

Less than 1% of American women between the ages of 20 and 39 suffer from coronary heart disease, according to a recent National Health and Nutrition Examination Survey. However, among 40- to 59-year-olds, that percentage climbs nearly 10-fold, to 5.6%. So, how can you stay healthy?

The name "cardio" is short for "cardiovascular," many people know that this form of heart-pumping exercise will keep the heart muscle robust;

o Running

o Spinning

o Dancing

o Rowing and

o Swimming

all count as cardio workouts.

However, if you really want your heart health to benefit from your cardio exercises, you need to exercise at 80% of your maximum heart rate for at least 30 minutes, 3 to 4 times a week. (On a scale of one to ten, with ten being as hard as you can push yourself, you should be around an 8.)

So, if you are hardly breaking a sweat while strolling or taking it easy during your favorite Zumba class, it is time to speed up your pace and boost your effort. Cardio workouts should seem effortful—like you could do it forever but would not want to."

2. High-Impact Activities (1 to 2 times a week)

Hint: This helps to ward off Osteoporosis

According to the National Osteoporosis Foundation, roughly 1 in 2 women over age 50 will break a bone because of osteoporosis, a condition in which the bones become brittle, increasing the risk of fractures.

Although you might be aware of calcium's role in maintaining a robust skeletal system, recent studies uncover additional insights, that high-impact, weight-bearing exercise can help build bone strength, too.

Despite the prevalent misconception that high-impact activities have more negative than positive effects, this is not accurate, especially concerning bone health.

o Dancing

o Jumping jacks

o Racquet sports

and even adding a moderate jog into your go-to walking regimen are all fantastic examples of exercise that can keep your bones strong.

3. Strength Training (2 to 3 times a week)

Hint: This helps to fight Arthritis

Strength or resistance training, which typically employs equipment such as weight machines, free weights, resistance bands, or tubing, protects against bone loss and builds muscle. It also enhances the proportion of lean muscle mass to fat in your body. It also merits a significant position in your workout regimen.

In technical terms, strength or resistance training occurs whenever your muscles encounter a force greater than usual, such as pushing against a wall or lifting a dumbbell.

Muscles become stronger through the use of increasingly heavier weights or heightened resistance. In addition to sculpting your physique, strength training furnishes the practical strength required for everyday tasks like lifting groceries, climbing stairs, getting up from a chair, and catching the bus effortlessly. The likelihood of developing arthritis rises as individuals age. Nevertheless, persistent joint discomfort and stiffness can affect adults of any age, particularly those who are overweight or have experienced a prior joint injury. Initiating the safeguarding of your body is a step that can be taken at any time.

Engaging in strength training stands out as an effective method to ward off discomfort and soreness. Research has demonstrated that engaging in strength training not only reduces arthritis-related pain but also serves as a preventive measure against its initial development. You don't have to dedicate extensive time in the weight room to enjoy the advantages.

All that's truly required is to engage in some type of:

o A squat

o Deadlift and

o Overhead press

these helps strengthen many joints and muscles.

4. Yoga (once a week)

Hint: This helps to battle Depression

Women between the ages of 45 and 64 have an elevated risk of depression, according to Johns Hopkins Medicine, one of the premier healthcare systems in the United States.

While any exercise can contribute to alleviating anxiety and depression, a growing body of research indicates that yoga may be especially advantageous in reducing stress and managing mood. A study revealed that yoga boosts levels of GABA, a neurotransmitter that regulates mood and is often deficient in individuals dealing with depression and anxiety. A different study discovered that women experiencing mental distress reported reduced stress levels after engaging in a three-month yoga program.

We know that yoga is amazing for stress reduction, and we know there's a correlation between stress and mood problems. Even better, certain kinds of yoga are also great weight-bearing strength training and even offer some cardiovascular conditioning, making it a win all around.

5. Plank (for 90 seconds, three times a week)

Hint: This helps to battle back pain

The National Institute of Arthritis and Musculoskeletal and Skin Diseases, part of The National Institutes of Health, reports that most individuals experience their initial bout of back pain between the ages of 30 and 40, with its frequency increasing as we age. To mitigate such pain, strengthening your core is crucial. The plant exercise is highly effective, targeting all core muscles including the abs, chest, and those surrounding the sine. This comprehensive workout not only tones your midsection but also provides essential support to your lower back, preventing pain.

To ensure proper form in the plank position, align your wrists under your elbows, position your elbows under your shoulders, and push the floor away with your feet.

Extend your legs behind you, keeping them shoulder-distance apart. Additionally, engage your abs by pulling your belly button towards your spine. Hold this position for 30 seconds, take a brief break on your knees, and then repeat the exercise twice more. As you build strength, aim to sustain the plank for 90 seconds without interruption.

Should you employ a personal trainer?
Hiring a personal trainer can surely bring added benefits when starting an exercise plan, as well as attending group fitness courses.

The benefit of a trained and experienced personal trainer or group teacher is having someone guide you through the right biomechanics, exercise selection, sequencing, intensity, and recuperation to enhance your results.

And if you add the community component that comes with group exercise, get ready to not only feel better physically but also mentally. A 2017 study in the Journal of the American Osteopathic Association found that people working out in a group setting resulted in lower stress levels and an improved quality of life compared to those working out alone.

Hiring a personal trainer or attending group sessions is also a smart method to avoid the "no pain, no gain" approach, which can lead to poor results, workout burnout, injury, or disease.

BEST ANTI-AGING EXERCISES YOU SHOULD TRY

1. SQUAT

Sets: 3 Reps: 10

If you want to stay young, perform squats! By doing so, you are working out the entire body – specifically, the hamstrings, the hips, the glutes, and the quads.

How to do it: To perform a squat, stand with your feet shoulder-width apart, then lower your hips down and back as if sitting in a chair. Keep your knees in line with your toes and your chest raised, and then stand back up.

Benefits of squats: Squats are one of the most effective exercises for building lower body strength, specifically targeting the glutes, quadriceps, and hamstrings in the legs. Squats can improve your balance and your level of coordination, stability, and bone density and reduce the risk of osteoporosis when done regularly.

2. LUNGES

Sets: 3 Reps: 10 on each leg

How to perform lunges: Begin by standing with your feet hip-width apart. Initiate a lunge by taking a substantial step forward with one foot, bending both knees until your back knee comes close to the ground. Push off the front foot to return to a standing position, then replicate the movement on the opposite side.

Advantages of lunges: Lunges are a lower-body exercise that can enhance strength and flexibility. They predominantly target the glutes, quadriceps, and hamstrings, while also engaging core muscles for stability.

3. DEADLIFTS

Sets: 3 Reps: 10

How to execute deadlifts: stand with your feet hp-width apart and position a barbell in front of you. Bend your knees and hinge at the hips to lower yourself and grasp the weight while maintaining a straight back. Rise back up lifting the weight using your legs and glutes, then lower it to the ground.

Advantages of deadlifts: Deadlifts are a comprehensive exercise that primarily targets the back muscles, glutes, and hamstrings. Additionally, they contribute to improved grip strength and overall mobility. If a barbell is unavailable, dumbbells can be used as an alternative for deadlifts.

4. OVERHEAD PRESSES

Sets: 3 Reps: 10

How to perform it: Begin by standing with your feet shoulder-width apart and the dumbbells resting on your upper chest. To keep your core engaged, press the dumbbells overhead by extending your arms straight up. To release slowly, start by bringing your elbows out to a 90-degree angle.

Benefits of overhead presses: The overhead press works the deltoids (your shoulder muscles) and is great at building strength in this area. It also engages the triceps and upper back muscles, making it a great move to improve the ability to do functional tasks such as placing an object on a high shelf or lifting a heavy suitcase.

5. PRESS-UPS

Sets: 3 Reps: 10

Begin in a plank position with your hands positioned shoulder-width apart and your feet spaced hip-width apart. Lower your body by bending your elbows, maintaining a straight line, and pushing back up to the starting position. For easier execution of the exercise, use an elevated surface like a bench or a sturdy couch to rest your hands on, or drop to your knees to lighten the load. Benefits of press ups: Press Ups are a basic workout that helps enhance upper body strength, notably targeting the chest, shoulders, and triceps. Additionally, push-ups activate the core muscles for stability and can improve total upper-body mobility.

6. PLANKS

Sets: 3 Time: 30 seconds

Assume a push-up position with hands and feet shoulder-width apart. Engage your core muscles to maintain a straight line from head to heels. your body stable. If you experience wrist joint pain, try performing this exercise on your elbows. How it helps: Planks are a core exercise that can improve general stability and posture and minimize the risk of back pain.

Planks target the abdominals, back muscles, and shoulder muscles, helping to enhance overall core strength.

7. STANDING CALF RAISE

Another anti-aging exercise that helps to reverse the natural aging process is the standing calf raise. This exercise targets the calf muscles – notably the one on the outer section of the leg that aids in shaping and setting the size of the calves.

8. HANGING LEG RAISE

Although challenging and requiring proper form, hanging leg raises are anti-aging exercises that target all core muscles.in your midsection and the lats. If you want to combat natural aging while building an immense amount of strength, this exercise will help you accomplish your goals.

9. WALKING

While it may seem to be a relatively ordinary exercise, walking is a weight-bearing activity that helps you—or, rather, forces you to work against the natural gravity that surrounds you. As a consequence, both your bones and muscles benefit. In turn, the overall performance of the complete body is optimized.

10. CLIMBING STAIRS

If you want to provide the lower section of your body with an intense workout, climb stairs! This activity engages all the muscles in your lower body. "This refers to the muscles located in the lower part of the body, specifically the calves, glutes, quadriceps, and hamstrings." As you progress with this exercise, your bones and joints will gain strength. As you age, performing this exercise can increase your endurance.

11. HIGH-IMPACT MOVEMENTS

While this is not a particular exercise, it is a type of movement that should be performed that is physical in nature. This is why it has made this list. Most experts recommend engaging in high-impact movements to reverse aging when exercising The actions I am referring to involve a combination of jumping, forceful stepping, and exaggerated movements when performed together. If you make certain that you perform high-impact movements on a daily basis, your bones will increase in density.

12. AEROBICS

"Do you feel uncomfortable at the idea of doing fast-paced aerobic exercise? " Not doing it will result in such a decline in health that it will make you cringe! This is a type of cardio exercise that will improve the health of your heart, your circulation, and your brain health – all of which are necessary to remain young!

13. RESISTANCE TRAINING

If you want to turn back the clock on your genes, resistance training is the way to do it! This sort of exercise boosts the strength of your muscles and optimizes your endurance level. You may accomplish it by integrating bands, weights, bars, dumbbells, and similar objects into your routine workout.

14. REACTION TRAINING

The second anti-aging exercise is response training. Examples include playing a sport such as tennis and indulging in Zumba. This improves your body, your reaction time, and your capacity to remember knowledge and change direction while maintaining your balance.

As a study published by the National Library of Medicine demonstrates, loss of muscle mass, decreased strength, and limited function are all common side effects of aging.

But the good news is a few simple lifestyle modifications can lessen the impact of aging and keep you limber for longer.

The more you exercise, the more you lengthen and strengthen your muscles, increasing your range of motion and preventing injuries. Consider adding yoga to your workout routine. Yoga is a great low-impact and low-intensity way to maintain mobility, strength, and flexibility as you age.

Effective Step-by-Step Anti-Aging Workout Routines: Enhancing Strength, Flexibility, and Balance

A good anti-aging workout regimen should focus on boosting strength, flexibility, and balance to help you maintain your general health and well-being as you age. Here's a step-by-step plan to construct a well-rounded fitness routine that addresses these crucial aspects:

Note: Before starting any new workout regimen, it's crucial to contact a healthcare practitioner, especially if you have any underlying health conditions or concerns.

Step 1: Warm-up (5-10 minutes)

Begin with a warm-up to boost blood flow, prepare your muscles, and lower the risk of injury. You can undertake activities like brisk walking, mild jogging, jumping jacks, or arm circles.

Step 2: Strength Training (2-3 times per week)

Strength training helps grow and maintain muscular mass, which can shrink with age. Focus on compound exercises that work for many muscle groups simultaneously. A sample routine might include:

1. Squats: 2-3 sets of 10-12 repetitions
2. Push-ups: 2-3 sets of 8-10 repetitions (adjust as needed)

3. Dumbbell Rows: 2-3 sets of 10-12 repetitions

4. Planks: 2 sets of 30-60 seconds

Gradually raise the weight or resistance over time to continue testing your muscles.

Step 3: Flexibility (2-3 times per week)

Maintaining flexibility is vital for preventing injury and maintaining a complete range of motion. Incorporate stretching activities, such as:

1. Neck stretches

2. Shoulder stretches

3. Leg stretches

4. Yoga or Pilates routines

To properly stretch your muscles, make sure to hold each stretch for 15 to 30 seconds, and repeat the process 2 to 3 times. Incorporate deep breathing to increase relaxation and flexibility.

Step 4: Balance (2-3 times each week)

Improving your balance will help reduce falls and injuries, which become increasingly common as we age. Try these balance-enhancing exercises:

1. Single-leg stands: Stand on one leg while lowering the other knee to hip level. Hold for 30 seconds, then switch legs. Do 2-3 sets for each leg.

2. Heel-to-toe walk: Walk in a straight line, placing one foot exactly in front of the other. Repeat for 20-30 feet.

3. Balance board exercises: Use a balance board or wobble board to challenge your balance further.

Step 5: Cardiovascular Exercise (3-5 times per week)

Cardiovascular exercise is crucial for general health and fitness. It helps enhance circulation, heart health, and stamina. Engage in activities like:

1. Brisk walking

2. Cycling

3. Swimming

4. Dancing

5. Aerobic classes

It is recommended that you engage in at least 150 minutes of moderate-intensity aerobic activity per week.

Step 6: Cool down and stretch for 5-10 minutes.

After your workout, cool down by walking or slowly jogging for a few minutes. Then, execute static stretches to release tension in the muscles. Focus on areas worked during your routine, such as the legs, arms, and back.

Step 7: Hydration and Nutrition

Staying hydrated and maintaining a balanced diet rich in lean proteins, fruits, vegetables, and whole grains is vital for general health and supporting your exercise.

Step 8: Rest and Recovery

Give your body time to recuperate between workouts. Adequate sleep, relaxation, and recovery days are vital for injury prevention and muscle restoration.

Remember to develop gradually, listen to your body, and make adjustments as needed. Consistency is crucial in any anti-aging fitness regimen. Additionally, consider working with a fitness professional or trainer to ensure that your routine matches your individual needs and goals.

Chapter 7

Beyond the Physical: Mind-Body Strategies for Agelessness

In the pursuit of eternal youth, unlocking the secrets to agelessness involves a holistic approach that incorporates not just physical routines but also taps into the profound connection between the mind and body. This chapter analyzes the profound influence of mind-body methods on the aging process and goes into the transforming worlds of mindfulness, meditation, and visualization as portals to agelessness.

Unveiling the Mind-Body Connection

Aging is not simply a physical phenomenon but also a cognitive and emotional one. The delicate interplay between the mind and body plays a vital role in how we feel the passage of time. Understanding and harnessing this mind-body connection is vital in our quest for agelessness.

The Power of Positive Thinking

Research suggests that maintaining a positive outlook might have a substantial impact on the aging process. Positive thoughts and attitudes can influence the release of neurotransmitters and hormones that contribute to general well-being. By fostering optimism and embracing a constructive attitude in life, individuals can potentially slow down the aging clock.

Mindfulness: A Pathway to Present Agelessness

The Essence of Mindfulness

Mindfulness entails being fully present in the current moment and appreciating the richness of each experience without judgment. As we age, our thoughts tend to concentrate on the past or worry about the future, contributing to stress and accelerating the aging process. Practicing mindfulness allows us to break out of this pattern and relish the beauty of the now.

Mindful Aging Practices

Incorporating mindfulness into everyday life can be a game-changer. Techniques such as mindful breathing, body scanning, and mindful movement not only boost mental clarity but also promote emotional resilience.

By accepting these activities, individuals can develop a foundation for agelessness by fostering a strong connection between the mind and body.

Meditation: Cultivating Inner Youthfulness
The Science of Meditation

Research has revealed that regular meditation can have dramatic benefits for the brain, boosting neuroplasticity and enhancing cognitive performance. These brain alterations can lead to a younger and nimbler mind, contradicting the prevalent assumptions about the inevitable deterioration of mental faculties with age.

Meditation Techniques for Agelessness

Explore diverse meditation approaches, such as mindfulness meditation, loving-kindness meditation, and transcendental meditation, to uncover the potential for agelessness. These techniques not only quiet the mind but also renew the body, promoting a harmonic balance between mental and physical well-being.

Visualization: Creating Your Ageless Reality
The Power of Visualization

Visualization includes forming mental representations of desired results and leveraging the mind's creative potential to materialize positive change. When applied to the quest for agelessness, visualization can be an effective tool for retraining the brain and affecting the body's responses to aging.

Ageless Living through Visualization

Guide readers through ageless living visualization exercises, urging them to see themselves in vigorous health, replete with energy and vitality. By constantly practicing these visualizations, individuals can modify their experience of aging and pave the way for a more youthful reality.

The Neuroplastic Symphony: Nurturing Cognitive Sharpness in Ageless Living

The science of neuroplasticity is a revelation that challenges the traditional wisdom about aging. It's a revelation that the brain is malleable, adaptive, and capable of creating new connections throughout life.

Neuroplasticity is the brain's response to experience, a symphony where neurons reorganize themselves in response to learning, challenges, and stimuli.

In the symphony of life, the brain leads the complex and complicated melodies that define our cognitive capacities. The concept of neuroplasticity, the brain's ability to reshape itself and generate new neural connections throughout life, has opened doors to a greater knowledge of how we may promote cognitive sharpness regardless of age. This voyage toward ageless life is analogous to orchestrating a neuroplastic symphony, where the harmonic interplay of diverse parts orchestrates the preservation and increase of cognitive function.

I. The Maestro Within: Understanding Neuroplasticity

1.1 The Adaptive Brain: Neuroplasticity is the brain's innate ability to adapt and restructure itself in response to experience, learning, and environmental changes. This phenomenon challenges the traditional view that the brain is a static organ, displaying its dynamic nature.

1.2 The Symphony of Neurons: Neurons are the instrumental performers in the neuroplastic symphony, forming connections termed synapses.

As we age, the brain's capacity to build new synapses and reinforce old ones becomes a vital determinant in preserving cognitive sharpness.

II. The Instruments of Ageless Cognition

2.1 Continuous Learning: Engaging in lifetime learning acts as a potent instrument in the neuroplastic symphony. Whether gaining a new skill, learning a language, or studying a new subject, the brain responds positively to unfamiliar challenges.

2.2 Physical Exercise: Exercise acts as the rhythmic beat in the neuroplastic symphony. Regular physical exercise has been related to the creation of neurotrophic factors, which stimulate the growth and survival of neurons, providing an environment conducive to neuroplasticity.

2.3 Nutritional Harmony: A balanced diet rich in antioxidants, omega-3 fatty acids, and other critical nutrients plays a vital role in promoting cognitive function. These nutritional nutrients operate as the sustaining notes that fortify the brain against the consequences of aging.

2.4 Adequate Sleep: The restorative power of sleep is the tranquil pause in the neuroplastic symphony.

During sleep, the brain consolidates memories, clears toxins, and enables synaptic plasticity, needed for healthy cognitive performance.

III. Conductor's Baton: Mindfulness and Stress Management

3.1 Mindfulness Meditation: Mindfulness meditation takes on the role of the conductor's baton, guiding attention and promoting a heightened awareness of the present moment. Studies suggest that mindfulness techniques can significantly alter brain structure and function, supporting neuroplasticity.

3.2 Stress as Dissonance: Chronic stress serves as discordant notes in the neuroplastic symphony, inhibiting cognitive function and accelerating brain aging. Stress management approaches, such as meditation and relaxation exercises, become vital in preserving cognitive sharpness.

IV. Technological Crescendo: Cognitive Training and Brain-Computer Interfaces

4.1 Cognitive Training: In the digital age, cognitive training programs employ technology to stimulate specific cognitive functions.

These applications operate as the technological instruments in the neuroplastic symphony, giving tailored workouts to boost memory, attention, and problem-solving skills.

4.2 Brain-Computer Interfaces (BCIs): As technology progresses, BCIs are emerging as a transformational force in the neuroplastic symphony. These interfaces permit direct contact between the brain and external devices, creating the potential for neurofeedback and cognitive development.

Tips for Ageless Living

Ageless existence does not take so much effort. Here's what you can do:

1. Maintain a Healthy Lifestyle: You can start following a regular and healthy schedule. You can add 30 minutes of exercise to your routine and eat a healthy and balanced diet. Plus, if you can avoid ingesting too much alcohol and smoking,

2. Nurture Social Connections: Try remaining in touch with people. In reality, you can invite others to social activities. You can go watch movies and indulge in activities with the ones you love.

Leading a happy and long life is easier if you have company and avoid loneliness.

3. Prioritize Mental Health: Another crucial thing you can do is keep your mind going toward new talents. You can get into reading, solving puzzles, or starting up a new pastime. The more your mind is engaged and your ideas are positive, the better your mental health will be. This can also assist you in lowering the risks of conditions like dementia.

4. Practice self-care: You can include meditation, breathing exercises, and relaxation techniques in your routine. You can even work toward obtaining enough sleep and minimizing stress levels. When you emphasize self-care, you will be able to have good health overall.

5. Embrace a Positive Attitude: Life has always thrown hurdles at us. "As one grows older, it becomes increasingly challenging." But, if you have a positive attitude toward life, complete with acceptance of what's going to occur and the ability to bounce back, you can lead a fantastic life. You would be able to offer your self-esteem a tremendous boost as well.

Chapter 8

Embracing the Art of Ageless Living

As we end our journey through the enthralling chapters of "How to Look Young in Old Age: Decoding the Science of Eternal Youth," we find ourselves standing at the intersection of science and wisdom, where the art of ageless living unfolds. Each chapter has been a step closer to deciphering the secrets of permanent youth, a trip that has brought us from the mystery of aging to the practical methods and techniques that pave the path to timeless beauty.

In Chapter 1, we dug into the great mystery of aging, studying the complicated science that underlies the process. **Chapter 2** exposed the ticking clock within us, revealing why our bodies succumb to the passage of time. The exploration proceeded in **Chapter 3** when we uncovered the figurative Fountain of Youth, an anti-aging toolbox loaded with formidable tools ready to be opened. Moving beyond theory, **Chapter 4** walks us through practical measures to reverse the hands of time, delivering a blueprint for timeless beauty.

We next stepped into the domain of nutrition in **Chapter 5**, discovering the ultimate anti-aging diet that nourishes not just the body but the very essence of perpetual youth.

Chapter 6 became a gym for the soul, shaping everlasting bodies via exercises suited for the ages.

Chapter 7 widened our horizons, investigating the profound relationship between mind and body and uncovering tactics that go beyond the physical. The combination of mind-body practices became a cornerstone for achieving agelessness, underscoring the need for holistic well-being.

Now, in this **final chapter**, we stand on the threshold of a new beginning—the culmination of knowledge, science, and the timeless wisdom that transcends the pages of this book. It is not just about defying the conventional restrictions of aging; it is about embracing a lifestyle that honors the art of ageless living.

As we bid farewell to the chapters that have unfolded like a gripping novel, let us carry with us the idea that age is not just a number but a canvas waiting to be painted with brilliant hues of health, energy, and joy. The voyage to perpetual youth is not a destination but a continuous investigation, a dance with the rhythm of life itself.

May this book be a guide and a partner in your search for ageless living? May it encourage you to face each day with the wonder of a child, the resilience of a warrior, and the knowledge of a sage. In the magnificent tapestry of life, let the chapters of your story remain perennially youthful, stitched with the threads of love, laughter, and a profound appreciation for the beauty that comes with the passage of time.

As we end this chapter, remember that the canvas of your life is still blank, awaiting the strokes of your choices, habits, and beliefs. Embrace the art of ageless life, for inside it lies the masterpiece of your perpetual youth.